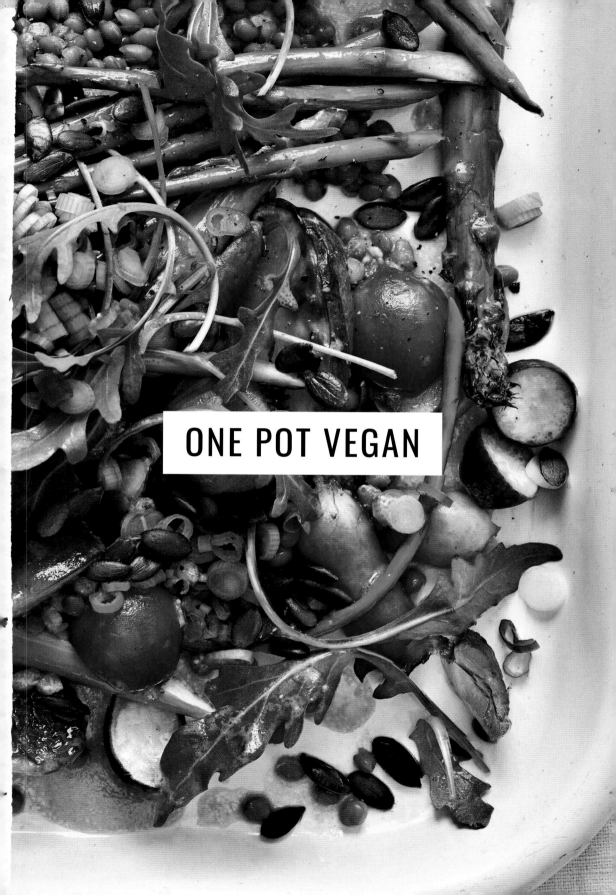

ONE POT VEGAN

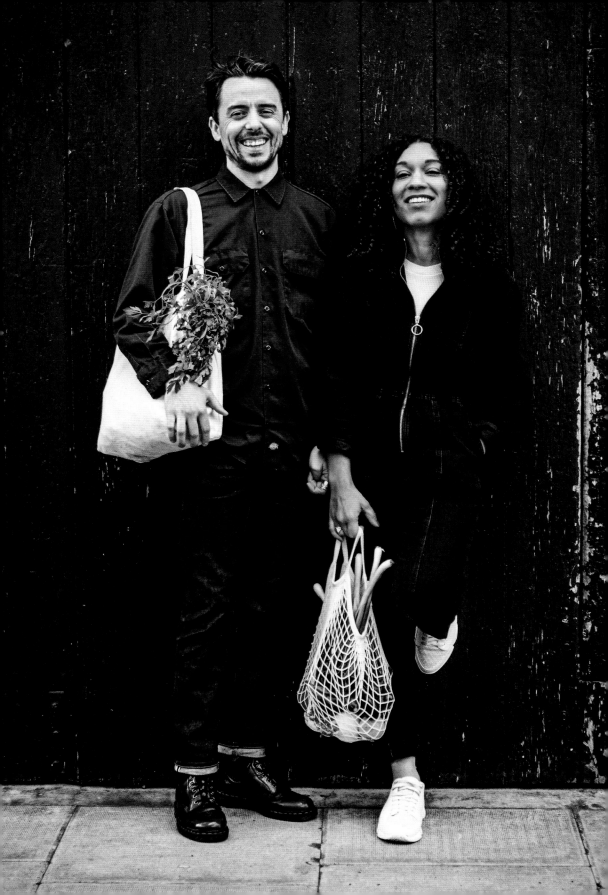

ONE POT VEGAN

80 quick, easy and totally delicious recipes.
Each using only one dish.

SO VEGAN

ROXY POPE + BEN POOK

michael joseph
an imprint of
penguin books

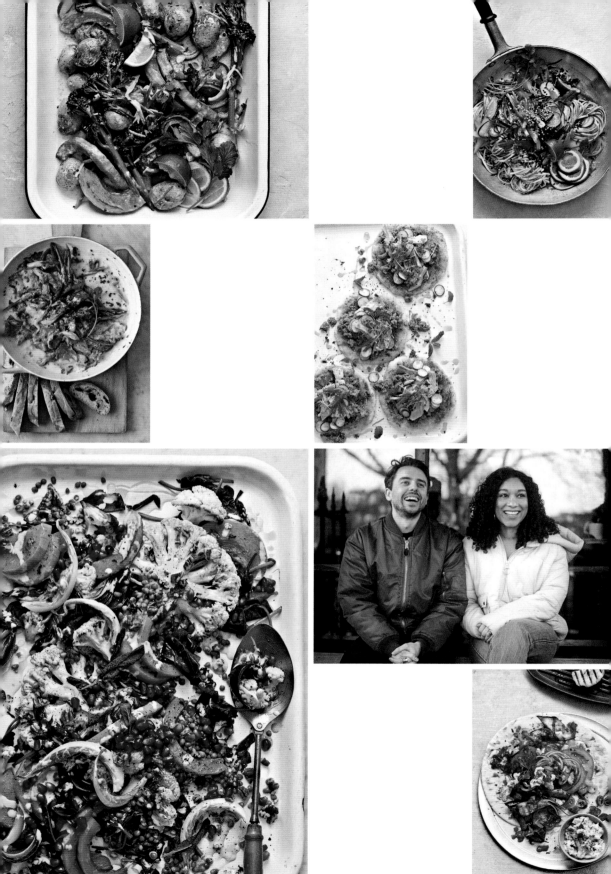

CONTENTS

INTRODUCTION

80 QUICK,
EASY +
TOTALLY
DELICIOUS
RECIPES.
EACH USING
ONLY ONE DISH.

If you're flicking through these pages wondering what you might want to rustle up for dinner tonight, the chances are we have something very important in common. We believe that **eating more plants is fundamentally a good thing**. Whether you think it's good for your health, good for the planet or good for animals – or possibly all three – getting more delicious plants on our plates can have a profoundly positive impact on our environment.

Our mission is simple: **we want to make it easy for everyone to eat more delicious plants so people and the planet can thrive**. This style of food shouldn't compromise on flavour. What's more, it doesn't have to be expensive or time-consuming. In fact it can be wonderfully quick and super easy. And that's exactly why we wanted to create *One Pot Vegan*.

Finding enough time in the day to cook delicious and nutritious meals can be tough! It often feels like we're living increasingly busier lives, and – if you're anything like the two of us – we bet you rarely find the time to do the stuff that really matters: catching up with old friends or diving into a new book.

The reality is . . . most of us simply don't have endless hours to spend in the kitchen. We also don't want to waste our time washing up countless pots and pans! So, in this book you will find 80 of our very best tried-and-tested recipes that use only one dish, whether it's a pot, a pan, a roasting tray or a cake tin. *One Pot Vegan* will make it easy for you and hopefully many others to eat more plants.

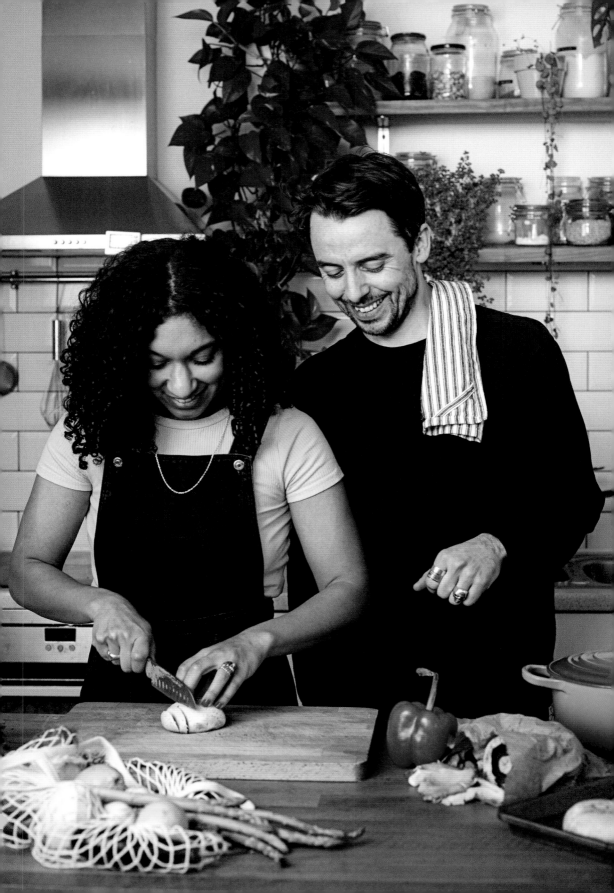

WE'VE CREATED THESE RECIPES FOR EVERYONE TO ENJOY, NOT JUST VEGANS

Maybe you follow us on social media or you're a regular visitor to our website. If so, thank you so much! If that is the case, then you'll know we're obsessed with creating 'veganized' versions of the classic dishes we grew up eating before we were vegan. You'll also know that So Vegan is a platform that welcomes everyone, whether you're vegan or simply curious about eating more plants.

This book is no different. *One Pot Vegan* is packed with one-pot, one-pan and one-tray recipes you'll want to cook again and again, designed for lifelong vegans and casual meat-eaters alike. Think of your favourite pastas, curries, salads, stir-fries, noodles and puddings, and there's a good chance we've created our very own version of it in this book. Our hope is that *One Pot Vegan* will be a reliable source of inspiration for your midweek meals and weekend feasts. From our rich, one-pan Lazy Lasagne (page 116) to our aromatic Aloo Gobi Traybake (page 80) and our insanely irresistible Crunchy Pecan & Cinnamon Sticky Buns (page 164), we've carefully developed these recipes to deliver **maximum flavour with minimum fuss**.

Writing this book was a huge challenge, but it was also an enormously rewarding experience. Everyday we were confronted with a host of unique problems we needed to solve. How on earth do we recreate a Chinese-inspired sweet and sour dish using only one tray, including the fluffy white rice? How about a one-pan veganized version of chicken supreme?

The truth is we've broken a lot of 'cooking traditions' creating this book! But this is precisely what makes these recipes so special to us. They're **our most innovative and exciting recipes yet**, and – most importantly – they're all developed to be incredibly simple for you to throw together in the comfort of your own kitchens.

We've also followed another simple rule: we only use ingredients we're able to find at our local supermarket. Some of these might be a little unfamiliar, and it may take you a few extra minutes to find them. But it was vital to us that we make everything as practical as possible. With that in mind, if you do struggle to find one or two of the ingredients in this book, **make sure you check out the 'tip' for each recipe**, where we probably suggest an easier-to-find substitute.

Hopefully we – and many other vegans – are living proof that you can absolutely thrive on a diet consisting only of plants. We genuinely feel as good as we ever have – both physically and mentally – and the food we love to eat every day is in this book. And yes, that also includes the occasionally indulgent treat! Following a diet which is good for your health is really important to us, which is why **we've included the nutritional information for all our recipes at the back**.

Before we forget, there are some other important things to know about *One Pot Vegan*. If you can, we recommend using a good-quality sea salt and freshly ground black pepper for seasoning. It's a relatively small expense and in return they'll deliver so much more flavour compared to slightly cheaper alternatives. We also wanted to stay as true to the concept of 'one pot' as possible, so there are only half a dozen or so occasions when we recommend using a food processor or a blender. We realize not everyone has a kitchen kitted out with these tools, so where possible we point out how to recreate these recipes without using extra equipment.

Well, that's about it! It's actually quite hard to put into words just how proud we are of this book and what it represents to us. More than anything else, creating this book has reminded us just how fortunate and privileged we are to do this for a living. Food has the power to transform people's lives – like it did ours – and to play just a small role in that feels very special. We really do hope you enjoy these fabulous recipes as much as we've enjoyed creating them for you.

Big love,

Roxy + Ben, aka So Vegan

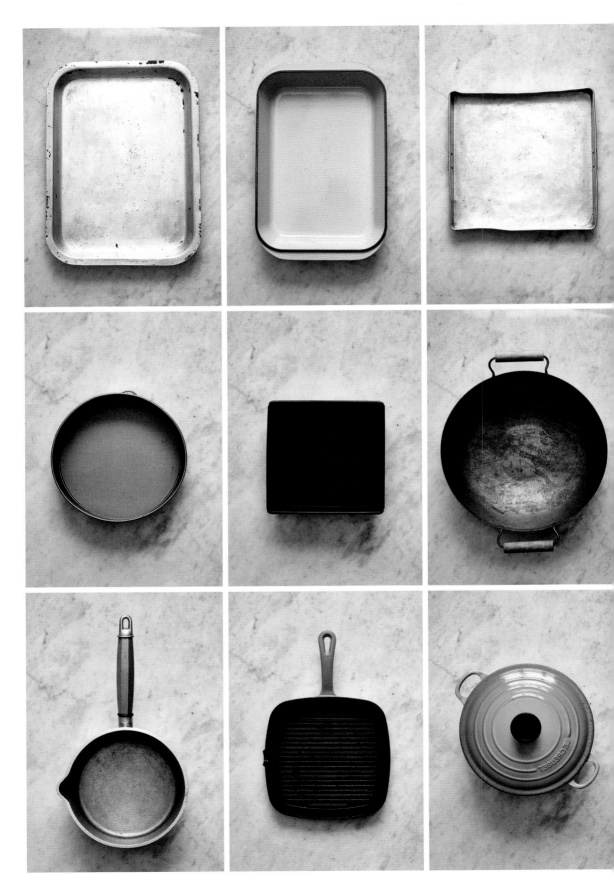

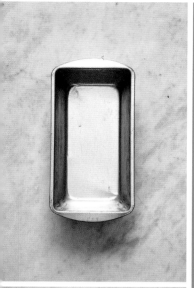

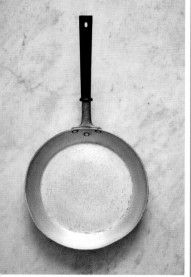

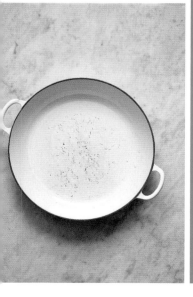

EQUIPMENT

'WE'RE BIG BELIEVERS IN MAKING THE MOST OF WHAT YOU'VE ALREADY GOT IN YOUR KITCHEN, WHETHER THAT'S THE FOOD IN YOUR FRIDGE OR THE POTS AND PANS PILED UP IN YOUR CUPBOARDS.'

The last thing we want to see is everyone rushing out to buy a brand-new casserole dish or a shiny new roasting tray when what you already own will probably do the trick.

At the top of every page we've included the pot, pan or tray we used to develop the recipe. We've tried really hard to keep the number of these different dishes down to a minimum, and you'll notice the same ones popping up throughout the book.

Like we said, it really isn't our intention to turn this into a shopping list. We've included specific measurements below, but honestly anything in these 'regions' will happily do and a few of our suggestions – such as the casserole pot and large saucepan – are sometimes interchangeable.

TRAYS + DISHES

Large roasting tray

Be prepared to get a lot of use out of this essential piece of kit. Roasting trays have raised sides and you'll need one at least a few centimetres deep for the likes of our Sweet & Sour Jackfruit (page 106), where we add water to the tray to cook the rice.

Our go-to roasting tray is 40cm x 30cm and it's ideal for the 'traybake' recipes in this book. If you're in the market for a new tray, don't forget to measure the size of your oven first! We once made this mistake and we now have a gigantic tray lying dormant in our cupboard.

Large baking tray

Similar to the above, anything close to 40cm x 30cm will cover all the baked goodies in this book. The flat sides will make it easier to remove the food from the tray, for example our Rhubarb & Frangipane Galette (page 166) and Mini Garden Flatbreads (page 42).

But to be honest, a large enough roasting tray will be sufficient – so as long as it's no more than a few centimetres deep.

Oven dish

The best thing about ovenproof dishes made of ceramic or glass is they'll keep your food warm for longer when out of the oven. This comes in particularly handy if you have lots of hungry people to feed around the dinner table, where it's often a lot easier to leave the food in the middle for everyone to help themselves.

Our dish is approximately 32cm x 22cm in size, and it's roughly 5cm deep. As always, anything in this region will work fine for the likes of our Sticky Buns (page 164) and Harissa Spiced Aubergines (page 114), so don't rush out to buy a new one if you don't have to.

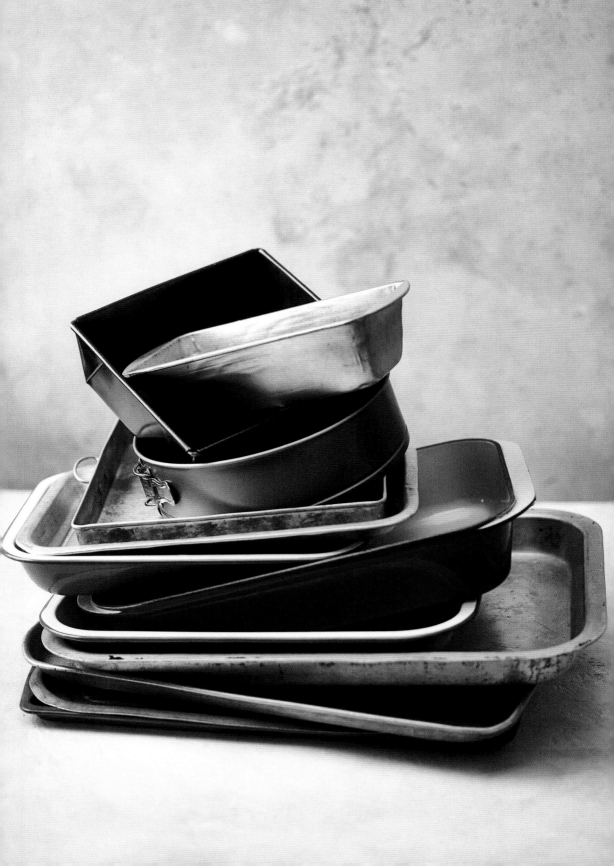

POTS

Casserole pot

This is our go-to piece of kit for curries, one-pot pastas and practically anything that requires some gentle 'stewing'. A good-quality casserole pot will have a thick base and sides, meaning it'll distribute heat more evenly. This also means it'll probably outlive you if you take good care of it.

We use a pot that is 24cm in diameter and 10cm deep, and it fits perfectly with the recipes in this book. Ours is also **ovenproof**, and this feature is put to good use for one of our recipes – the Smoky Sausage Cassoulet (page 124) – where we transfer the pot from the stovetop to the oven.

Large saucepan

A large saucepan will come in handy for a couple of our pasta recipes. This is where we keep things super simple, such as boiling the pasta and simmering the sauce. Use a saucepan that will fit enough pasta for four people and you'll be on the right track. Ours is roughly 20cm in diameter and 10cm deep, and of course there's no harm in using a similar-sized casserole pot.

TINS

Loose-bottomed cake tins

The truth is we've lost count of the number of cake tins we now own in various shapes and sizes. Most of them go unused because we always turn to our trusted favourites, including our loose-bottomed round cake tin, which is 20cm in diameter. It makes quick work of removing our Cardamom & Pistachio Shortbread (page 174) and Upside Down Cake (page 168) from their tins!

We prefer to slice our Brownies (page 156), Blondies (page 158) and Crumb Cake (page 159) into squares, which is where our 20cm x 20cm loose-bottomed square cake tin is put to work. But don't go to the effort of buying a square tin when a round version will do, and vice versa. We've never heard anyone complain about round brownies or blondies!

Loaf tin

A sturdy loaf tin is a kitchen staple. You'll need a large '2lb' sized version, which works out at roughly 25cm x 13cm x 7cm, for our Boozy Caribbean Pear Cake (page 170). These wonderful vessels are also more versatile than lots of people think, and are great for fruitcake, nut roast, and, of course, homemade bread!

PANS

Frying pan

Any regular-sized frying pan will do the job. We use a combination of stainless steel and non-stick frying pans. 'Non-stick' pans don't always have a great reputation, but if the pan is of a decent quality and you take reasonable care of it, then it'll be worth the modest investment.

Our pans are mostly 28cm in diameter, which leaves plenty of room for our Kofte Kebabs (page 94) and vegan 'Fishcakes' (page 108).

Wok

Our trusted wok is a lifesaver when it comes to stir-frying veggies. The design of a wok helps to distribute heat more evenly and – most importantly – prevents the food ending up all over the floor when it tumbles all over itself.

It's also important to avoid overcrowding your veggies in a wok so they cook evenly, so our Udon Noodles (page 64) and Rainbow Noodles (page 32) are designed to serve two. But don't rush out to buy a new wok if you don't want to – a regular frying pan will do.

Shallow casserole pan

We found ourselves reaching for our shallow casserole pan again and again while writing this book. Whether we're cooking Risotto (page 71), Paella (page 138) or Lazy Lasagne (page 116), the thick base and sides – much like our casserole pot – are far better at distributing heat compared to a regular pan.

A casserole pan which is anything close to 26cm in diameter and 5cm deep will treat you well as you navigate your way through this book. Just keep an eye out for a few recipes which require an **ovenproof** version, including our Mushroom & Ale Pie (page 150), which has a flaky filo top.

Griddle pan

Is a griddle pan completely necessary? No, definitely not – and you'll easily get by without one. But it'll come in handy for a couple of our recipes – Aubergine Kebabs (page 120) and Grilled Fruits (page 162) – if you want to capture that 'charred' flavour.

LIGHTS

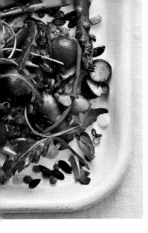

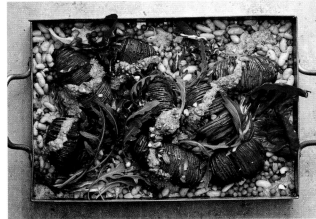

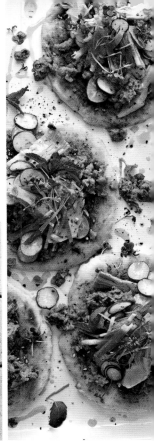

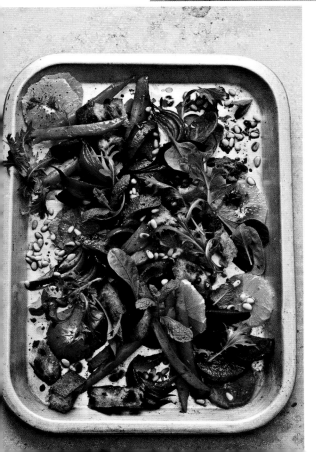

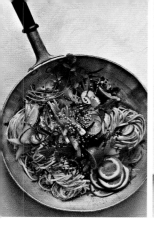
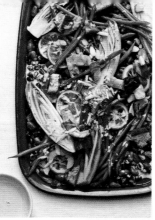
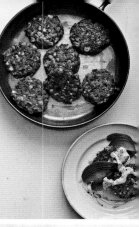

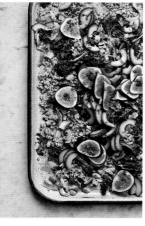
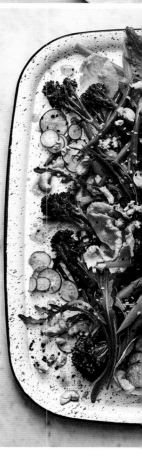
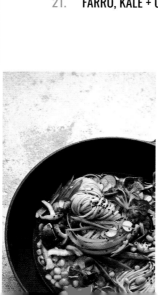

ROASTED BEETROOT + ORANGE SALAD

If there's one thing that unites us more than anything else, it's our shared and unconditional love of beetroot. Here we balance its earthy flavour with fresh, tangy orange.

SERVES 3–4   **DISH** LARGE ROASTING TRAY   **PREP** 25 MINS   **COOK** 40 MINS

6 medium beetroots (600g)

4 medium carrots (400g)

2 red onions

1½ tbsp maple syrup

½ tbsp dried oregano

½ tbsp fennel seeds

1 tbsp sumac

½ tbsp ground cumin

salt and pepper

olive oil

220g crusty bread (we use one with nuts and raisins)

3 tbsp pine nuts

1½ tbsp balsamic vinegar

extra virgin olive oil

2 oranges

20 fresh mint leaves

2 handfuls of mixed salad leaves (watercress, rocket and spinach)

Preheat the oven to 200°C fan/220°C/gas 7. Peel the beetroots and slice into eighths. Slice the carrots into batons, and quarter the red onions, leaving the skins on both. Transfer all to a large roasting tray, pour over the maple syrup, sprinkle over the oregano, fennel seeds, sumac, cumin, 1 teaspoon of salt and a large pinch of pepper. Pour over 2 tablespoons of olive oil and mix everything together.

Roast for 30 minutes, stirring halfway through. Meanwhile, cut the bread into 2cm cubes.

Remove the tray from the oven, pick out the red onions and save them for later, discarding the skins. Sprinkle over the bread and pine nuts, then return the tray to the oven for a final 10 minutes. Take the tray out of the oven again and put the roasted red onion back in. Pour over 1 tablespoon of balsamic vinegar and give everything a good mix, then leave the veggies to cool slightly while you complete the next steps.

In a small bowl, combine 2 tablespoons of extra virgin olive oil with the remaining ½ tablespoon of balsamic vinegar, a pinch of salt and pepper, and the zest from half an orange. Stir to combine.

Top and tail the oranges. Stand the oranges upright on one of their cut ends on a chopping board. Remove the skins and pith in strips by cutting from top to bottom, following the curve of the orange. Then slice the oranges into 1cm-thick circles. Roughly chop most of the mint leaves, leaving a few for decorating.

Scatter the mixed salad leaves, sliced oranges and chopped mint over the veggies, then pour over the dressing. Give everything a good stir, then top with the remaining mint leaves. Yum!

We often substitute the pine nuts with walnuts, to keep costs down.

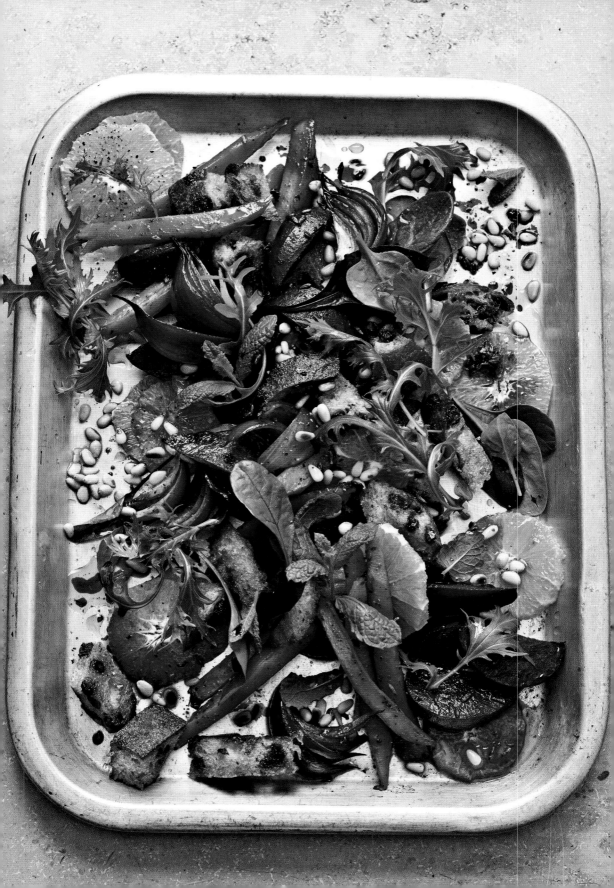

TANGY ROASTED FENNEL + BULGUR SALAD

Roasted fennel is hard to beat. You end up with a wonderfully soft texture and a caramelized sweetness, while preserving a subtle anise-like flavour.

SERVES 4 **DISH** LARGE ROASTING TRAY **PREP** 10 MINS **COOK** 45 MINS

3 fennel bulbs,
   with fronds still
   attached (900g)

350g cherry
   tomatoes

salt and pepper

1 tbsp mustard seeds

olive oil

250g bulgur wheat

500ml vegetable
   stock

100g chopped kale

80g walnuts

80g radicchio

1 lemon

2 tsp Dijon mustard

2 tsp maple syrup

extra virgin olive oil

Preheat the oven to 180°C fan/200°C/gas 6. Trim and quarter the fennel, saving the green fronds for garnish. Transfer to a large roasting tray with the cherry tomatoes. Sprinkle over ½ teaspoon of salt, a large pinch of pepper and the mustard seeds, then drizzle over 1 table-spoon of olive oil. Give everything a good mix and roast in the oven for 25 minutes.

Remove the tray from the oven and add the bulgur (try to fill in the gaps around the tray and avoid scattering it over the veggies). Then add the vegetable stock along with 100ml of hot water, making sure the bulgur is submerged in the liquid. Carefully return the tray to the oven for 15 minutes.

Take the tray out of the oven, fluff the bulgur up a little with a fork, and scatter the kale and walnuts on top of the veggies. Return the tray to the oven for 5 minutes, until the kale starts to crisp at the edges.

Meanwhile, roughly chop the radicchio. Next prepare the vinaigrette by grating the zest from the lemon into a small jug, then add the juice from the lemon, the Dijon mustard, maple syrup, 3 tablespoons of extra virgin olive oil and pinches of salt and pepper. Give it all a good stir.

Remove the tray from the oven for the final time and stir in the radicchio. Then drizzle over the vinaigrette, sprinkle over the green fronds and serve. Lush!

> Any type of crunchy lettuce will work here in place of radicchio.

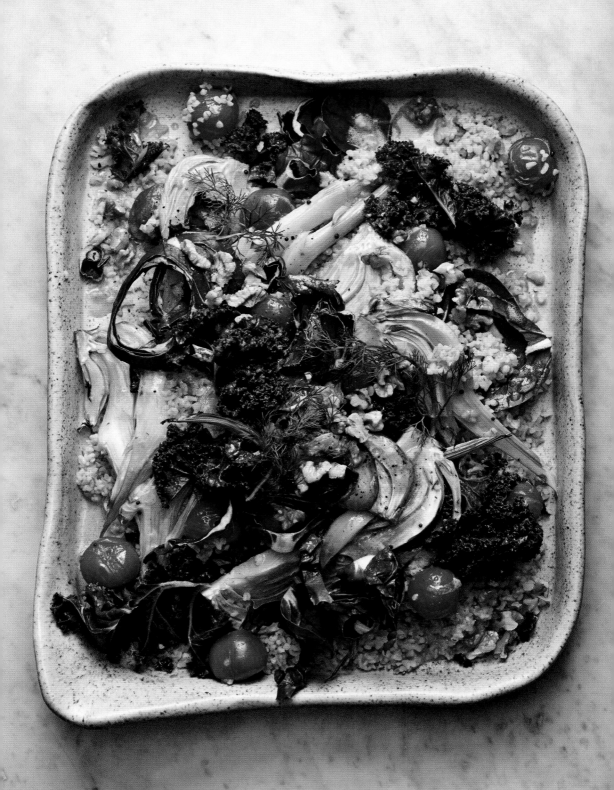

FIERY CHIPOTLE FRITTERS

Brunch? Snack? Dinner? These fritters have you covered. The chickpea flour binds everything together, while the chipotle paste gives these delicious patties a warm and smoky kick.

MAKES 10 FRITTERS   **DISH** FRYING PAN   **PREP** 15 MINS   **COOK** 45 MINS

3 medium courgettes (600g)

200g fresh corn kernels (or frozen sweetcorn)

4 spring onions

a handful of fresh coriander (15g)

100g chickpea (gram) flour

1 tbsp chipotle paste

1 tsp dried oregano

1 tsp dried thyme

salt and pepper

olive oil

1 avocado, for serving (optional)

vegan crème fraîche, for serving (optional)

Coarsely grate the courgette, then put it into a clean tea towel and squeeze out as much liquid as possible over a sink. Transfer the courgette to a mixing bowl along with the corn kernels (if using frozen, first rinse them in a sieve under cold water until thawed).

Thinly slice the spring onions. Pick the coriander leaves off their stalks and roughly chop them. Add both to the mixing bowl, followed by the chickpea flour, chipotle paste, oregano, thyme, 1 teaspoon of salt and a large pinch of pepper. Combine everything together with your hands, making sure the chipotle paste is dispersed evenly throughout the mixture. Add more chickpea flour if the mixture is too wet.

Put 2 tablespoons of olive oil into a frying pan over a low-medium heat. As soon as the oil is hot, take a tenth of the mixture and compact it into a round fritter using your hands, then add it to the pan. Repeat quickly until you have 3–4 fritters in the pan, then cover and fry for 6–8 minutes on each side, until crispy and cooked through. Be careful when you remove the lid, as moisture may cause the oil to spit. Repeat, wiping out any bits from the pan and adding a splash more oil, if needed, until you've cooked all the fritters.

Cut the avocado in half, remove the stone, scoop out the flesh and slice. Serve the fritters with the sliced avocado and vegan crème fraîche. Deeelicious.

You're most likely to find chickpea flour, aka gram flour, in the world foods section at your local supermarket.

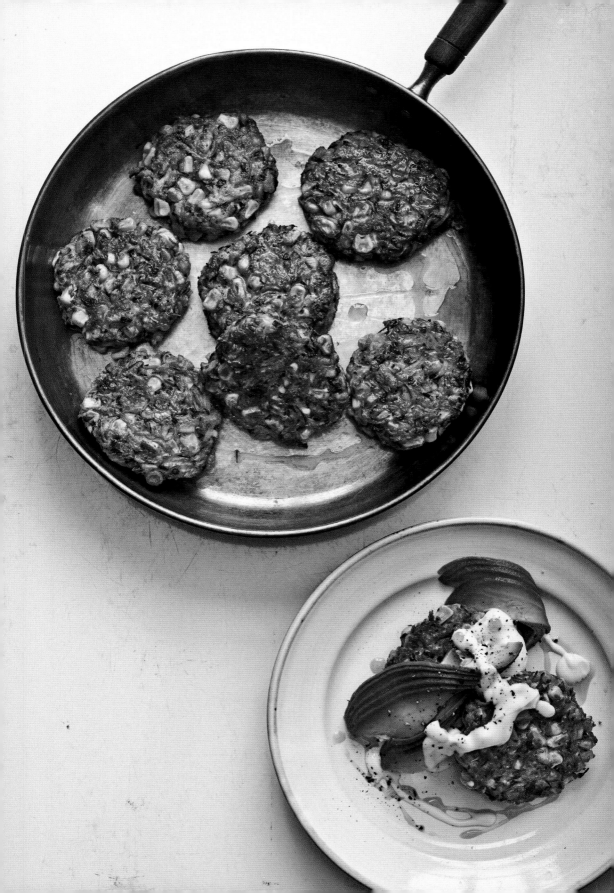

SPRING GREEN SALAD

There's something undeniably satisfying about eating fresh and seasonal produce. This simple light salad is made for those early sun-soaked days.

SERVES 4   **DISH** LARGE ROASTING TRAY   **PREP** 15 MINS   **COOK** 30 MINS

1kg new potatoes

6 shallots

salt and pepper

olive oil

300g asparagus spears

250g radishes

1 x 400g tin of green lentils

4 tbsp pumpkin seeds

extra virgin olive oil

1 lemon

1 tbsp Dijon mustard

½ tbsp maple syrup

a large handful of fresh dill (20g)

2 spring onions

2 handfuls of rocket

Preheat the oven to 220°C fan/240°C/gas 9. Cut any larger potatoes in half. Peel the shallots and cut in half, then put both into a large roasting tray, season with salt and pepper, and drizzle with 2 tablespoons of olive oil. Toss with your hands, then roast for 20 minutes.

Trim the woody ends off the asparagus. Cut the asparagus and radishes in half, add to the baking tray, drizzle with 1 tablespoon of olive oil and sprinkle with salt and pepper. Toss everything with a metal spoon and roast for 5 minutes.

Drain and rinse the lentils, then add them to the baking tray along with the pumpkin seeds and roast for 5 minutes.

Remove the tray from the oven. For the dressing, combine 2 tablespoons of extra virgin olive oil with the juice of the lemon, the Dijon mustard, maple syrup and pinches of salt and pepper.

Finely chop the dill and spring onion, then sprinkle over the salad along with the rocket. Pour the dressing over everything and toss to combine. All done!

> Reinvent this recipe by swapping the pumpkin seeds and lentils for any other seed and pulse.

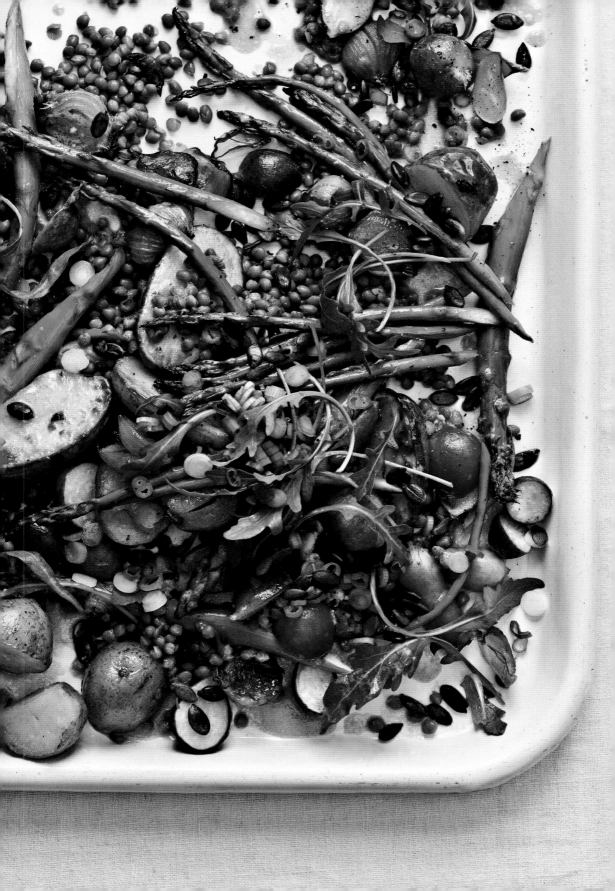

OUR GO-TO RAMEN

In 2012 we cycled from Kyoto all the way to Tokyo, sustaining ourselves on some of the finest ramen in the world. To this day we still enjoy filling our bellies with this tasty hot broth.

SERVES 2   **DISH** WOK   **PREP** 15 MINS   **COOK** 15 MINS

200g mixed wild mushrooms

1 shallot

2 garlic cloves

½ a thumb of fresh ginger (15g)

vegetable oil

800ml vegetable stock

½ tbsp brown rice miso paste

½ tsp chilli oil, plus extra for serving

100g wholewheat noodles

80g frozen edamame

80g frozen sweetcorn

80g mangetout

sesame oil

To top with (optional):

a handful of radishes

½ a carrot

a handful of lamb's lettuce

2 tsp sesame seeds

Trim the large mushrooms into smaller pieces, then peel and chop the shallot, garlic and ginger. Heat 2 tablespoons of vegetable oil in a wok on a medium-high heat. Once hot, fry the mushrooms, shallots, ginger and garlic for 5 minutes.

Add the vegetable stock, miso paste, chilli oil and noodles, bring to the boil, then reduce the heat and simmer for 5 minutes. Meanwhile, thinly slice the radishes and cut the carrot into matchsticks.

Add the edamame, sweetcorn and mangetout to the ramen and cook for 3–5 minutes, or until the noodles are cooked and the veggies are slightly tender. Stir in a drizzle of sesame oil and top with the sliced radishes, carrot, lamb's lettuce, a drizzle of extra chilli oil and a sprinkling of sesame seeds.

> Mixed wild mushrooms add a lovely variety of textures and flavour, but any mushrooms will do.

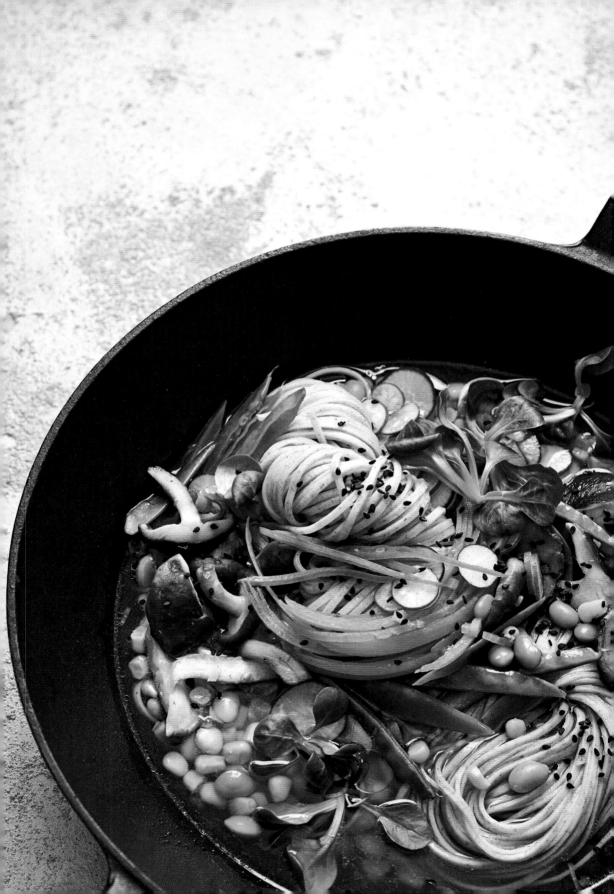

LOADED SWEET POTATO WEDGES

A celebration of the humble sweet potato. Here we roast them as wedges, as well as blend them to create our very own homemade queso. Delish.

SERVES 2–4   **DISH** LARGE ROASTING TRAY   **PREP** 20 MINS   **COOK** 45 MINS

50g cashews

1.2kg sweet potatoes

salt and pepper

vegetable oil

2 red onions

3 garlic cloves

1 ripe mango

1 red pepper

a handful of fresh coriander (15g), plus extra for topping

1 lime

2 x 400g tins of black beans

1 tbsp Cajun seasoning

4 tbsp nutritional yeast

180ml unsweetened plant-based milk

1 red chilli

1 avocado

Preheat the oven to 200°C fan/220°C/gas 7. Put the cashews into a bowl, cover with hot water from the kettle, and set to one side to soak.

Dice 200g of the sweet potatoes into 1cm pieces and place in the corner of a large roasting tray. Slice the remaining sweet potatoes into wedges, then place at the other end of the tray. Season the wedges with ½ teaspoon of salt and a large pinch of pepper, drizzle over 2 tablespoons of vegetable oil, and toss to combine. Slice 1 red onion in half, skin on, and add it to the tray along with the garlic cloves (skins on). Roast for 20 minutes.

For the salsa, cut the mango in half around the stone, slice the halves in a criss-cross pattern and scoop out the cubes of mango. Dice the red pepper, discarding the core and the seeds. Peel and dice the remaining red onion and roughly chop the coriander leaves, discarding the stalks. Add everything to a mixing bowl along with the juice from half the lime, and a pinch of salt and pepper. Mix everything together.

Take the tray out of the oven and remove the onion, garlic cloves and diced sweet potato to use later. Move the sweet potato wedges around the tray, then return the tray to the oven for 10 minutes.

Drain and rinse the black beans. Add them to the tray along with the Cajun seasoning and gently give everything a mix. Roast for 10–15 minutes, or until the sweet potato is lightly charred.

To make the queso, drain the cashews and transfer them to a high-powered blender or food processor, along with the diced sweet potato, roasted red onion and garlic (skins removed from both), nutritional yeast, juice from the remaining lime half, milk, half the red chilli (seeds removed), and large pinches of salt and pepper. Blend until smooth.

Remove the wedges from the oven and scatter over the salsa and half the queso. Thinly slice the remaining chilli and roughly chop the rest of the coriander leaves. Cut the avocado in half, scoop out and slice the flesh, then add it to the wedges, along with the sliced chilli and coriander leaves. Serve alongside the remaining queso. Epic.

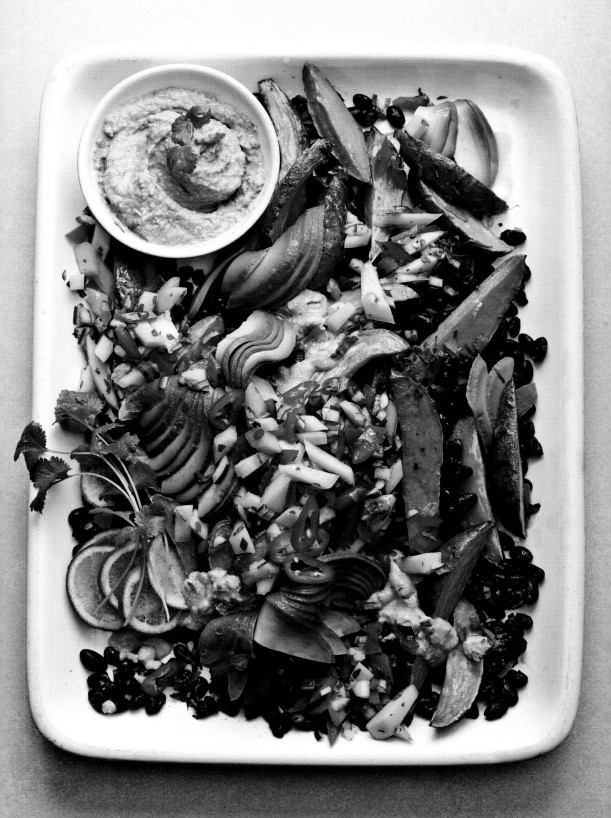

RAINBOW NOODLES

'Eat the rainbow.' It's often as simple as that. If you eat lots of different-coloured fruits and veggies, the chances are you'll be consuming a variety of vitamins and nutrients. Win.

SERVES 2　**DISH** WOK　**PREP** 15 MINS　**COOK** 8–11 MINS

½ a thumb of fresh ginger (15g)

150g red cabbage

1 medium carrot

1 red chilli

a large handful of fresh mint (20g)

a large handful of fresh coriander (20g)

8 radishes

½ a ripe mango

3 tbsp sesame seeds

vegetable oil

300g straight-to-wok noodles

salt

½ a lime

For the hoisin sauce:

4 tbsp raisins

2 tsp maple syrup

1 tbsp light soy sauce

1 tbsp apple cider vinegar

½ tsp Chinese five spice

½ tbsp sesame oil

Put the raisins into a small bowl and cover with 4 tablespoons of hot water from the kettle. Leave to one side for the raisins to soften.

Next prepare the veggies. Peel and chop the ginger. Thinly slice the red cabbage, slice the carrot into thin batons (keep the nutritious skin on) and slice the chilli (keep the seeds if you prefer things spicy). Pick the mint and coriander leaves off their stalks, and thinly slice the radishes. Then slice the flesh from the mango half into strips.

Place a wok on a medium-high heat and lightly toast the sesame seeds for 2–3 minutes, then transfer them to a small bowl. Place the wok back on the heat and add 1 tablespoon of vegetable oil. As soon as the oil is hot, add the ginger, red cabbage and carrot and fry for 3–4 minutes, stirring frequently.

Transfer the raisins and their soaking water to a fast-powered blender (see tip below if you don't have a blender). Add the remaining hoisin sauce ingredients and blend until smooth (alternatively you can use a hand-held blender). Pour the sauce into the wok and fry for 2 minutes, stirring frequently.

Add the sliced radishes, chilli and mango, a pinch of salt, the juice from the lime half, most of the fresh herbs and most of the toasted sesame seeds to the wok, give everything a good stir, then keep stirring and frying for 1–2 minutes. Finally, add the noodles and stir until warmed through. Top with the remaining herbs and toasted sesame seeds to serve.

> If you don't have a blender, simply chop the raisins and add them straight to the wok along with the remaining ingredients for the hoisin sauce.

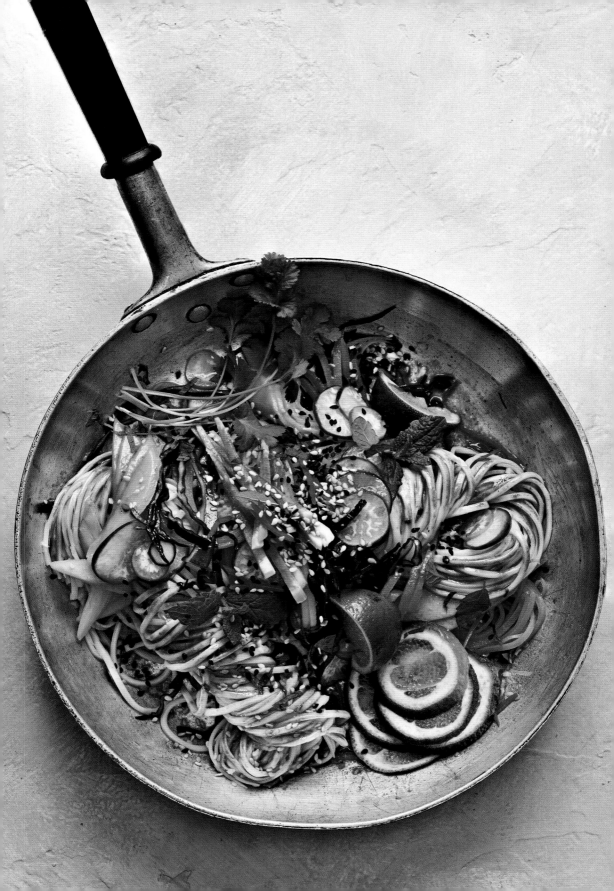

ROASTED PARSNIP + CRISPY PITTA FATTOUSH

Originating in Lebanon, fattoush is a simple, colourful salad enjoyed throughout the Middle East, and it happens to pair brilliantly with crispy roasted parsnips.

SERVES 4   **DISH** LARGE ROASTING TRAY   **PREP** 15 MINS   **COOK** 45 MINS

5 medium parsnips (500g)

olive oil

1 tbsp maple syrup

1 tbsp sumac, plus 1 tsp

salt and pepper

4 pittas

100g fresh flat-leaf parsley

a bunch of fresh mint (30g)

3 spring onions

½ a large cucumber (200g)

300g cherry tomatoes (we use a variety of colours)

10 radishes

1 garlic clove

½ a lemon

extra virgin olive oil

Preheat the oven to 180°C fan/200°C/gas 6. Trim the ends off the parsnips and slice them into quarters lengthways. Transfer to a large roasting tray, drizzle over 2 tablespoons of olive oil and the maple syrup, and sprinkle over 1 tablespoon of sumac and a pinch of salt and pepper. Give everything a mix and roast for 20 minutes.

Meanwhile, slice the pittas into 4cm squares and transfer to a bowl. Drizzle over 1 tablespoon of olive oil, and sprinkle over ½ teaspoon of sumac and a small pinch of salt and pepper. Give everything a good mix.

Remove the tray from the oven and add the pitta squares. Mix everything together, then return to the oven for another 15 minutes.

Roughly chop the parsley and mint leaves, discarding the stalks (save a few mint leaves for topping). Thinly slice the spring onions, roughly dice the cucumber, halve the cherry tomatoes and thinly slice the radishes, discarding the tough ends.

Remove the tray from the oven and mix in the chopped veggies and herbs.

Prepare a simple dressing: peel and finely chop the garlic, and put it into a small jug along with the juice of half a lemon, 2 tablespoons of extra virgin olive oil and a small pinch of salt and pepper. Stir to combine. Finally sprinkle ½ teaspoon of sumac over the parsnip fattoush, top with the remaining mint leaves and serve with the dressing.

> Dig around for any leftover root veggies lying at the back of the fridge – they can be put to good use along with the parsnips in this fattoush.

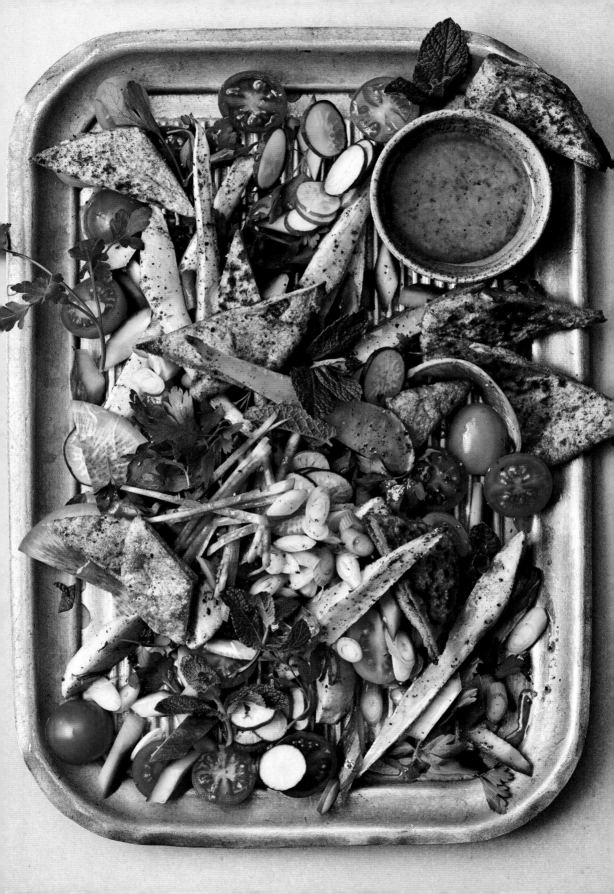

BLACK DHAL

Dhal is so much more than just a lentil curry. It's found on practically every dinner table in India, and for our black dhal we add a bounty of spices to give it that comforting kick.

SERVES 4   **DISH** CASSEROLE POT   **PREP** 15 MINS   **COOK** 70 MINS

1 onion

2 tbsp vegan
   margarine

6 garlic cloves

a thumb of fresh
   ginger (30g)

2 red chillies

1½ tbsp ground
   cumin

1 tbsp ground
   coriander

2 tsp garam masala

½ tsp ground
   cinnamon

1½ tsp mustard
   seeds

400g beluga lentils

1 x 400g tin of plum
   tomatoes

1 litre vegetable
   stock

2 tbsp tomato purée

salt and pepper

150ml vegan single
   cream

a handful of fresh
   coriander (15g)

4 vegan naans

Peel and finely dice the onion. Put 1 tablespoon of margarine into a casserole pot on a medium heat. Once the pan is hot, fry the onion for 8–10 minutes, until golden and translucent.

Meanwhile, peel and chop the garlic and ginger and finely chop one of the chillies (leaving the seeds in). Add to the pot along with the spices and fry for 2 minutes. Add extra margarine if it's too dry.

Rinse the lentils until the water runs clear, then drain. Add them to the pot along with the tinned tomatoes, stock, tomato purée and generous pinches of salt and pepper. Bring the dhal to the boil, then reduce the heat and simmer with the lid on for 50–70 minutes, or until the lentils are super soft and the dhal is nice and thick. Stir occasionally, and add water, a few tablespoons at a time, if it gets too dry. Taste and season with extra salt and pepper as needed.

Stir in 100ml of the vegan single cream and 1 tablespoon of margarine. Drizzle the rest of the vegan cream on top, then finely slice the remaining chilli and sprinkle over the dhal. Pick the coriander leaves off their stalks and scatter them over the top, then warm the naans in a toaster or microwave and serve.

> Beluga lentils can be found in the world foods aisle at your local supermarket. You can also sub them with green, brown or Puy lentils instead.

TRAYBAKE MUJADARA + PARSLEY SALAD

Mujadara is a medieval Arab dish originating in Iraq. Traditionally cooked over a stove, this combination of simple and humble ingredients works just as well roasted in an oven.

SERVES 4 **DISH** LARGE ROASTING TRAY **PREP** 15 MINS **COOK** 35 MINS

3 onions

olive oil

1 tbsp ground cumin

2 tsp ground coriander

salt and pepper

1 x 400g tin of green lentils

250g bulgur wheat

500ml vegetable stock

3 tomatoes (270g)

½ a large cucumber (200g)

a bunch of fresh flat-leaf parsley (30g)

extra virgin olive oil

200g vegan plain yoghurt

Preheat the oven to 200°C fan/220°C/gas 7. Peel and thinly slice the onions. Put them into a large roasting tray and drizzle over 2 tablespoons of olive oil, then add the cumin, coriander, ½ teaspoon of salt and 1 teaspoon of pepper. Give everything a mix, spread the onions out evenly on the tray, then bake for 16–18 minutes, stirring the onions halfway through to make sure they cook evenly.

Remove a third of the onion and leave it to one side. Reduce the oven temperature to 180°C fan/200°C/gas 6. Drain and rinse the lentils, then add them to the tray along with the bulgur wheat. Give everything a good mix, then pour over the stock and top up with 100ml of hot water. Mix again, making sure the bulgur is distributed evenly in the tray, then return to the oven for 15–20 minutes, stirring everything halfway through.

Meanwhile, dice the tomatoes and cucumber, and pick the parsley leaves off their stalks. When the mujadara is ready, top with the diced tomato, cucumber, parsley leaves, reserved crispy onions and an extra sprinkle of freshly ground black pepper. Serve with a drizzle of extra virgin olive oil and dollops of the vegan yoghurt. Superb.

> Box up any leftovers for lunch the next day. This mujadara will store well for at least a day in the fridge.

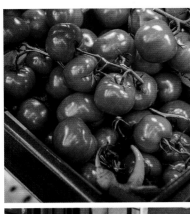
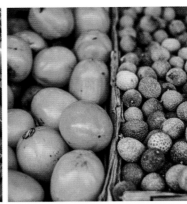
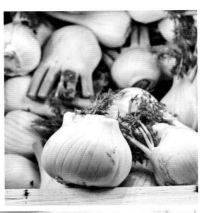
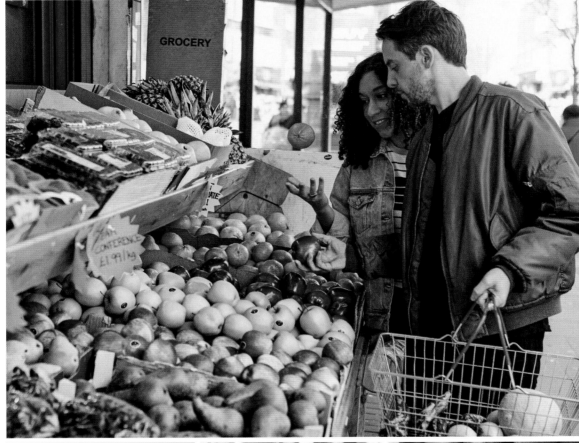
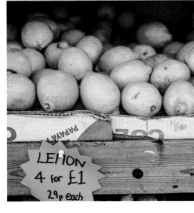
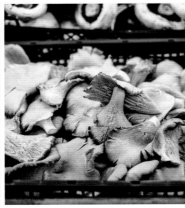
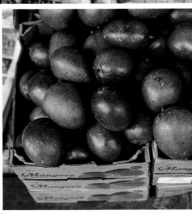

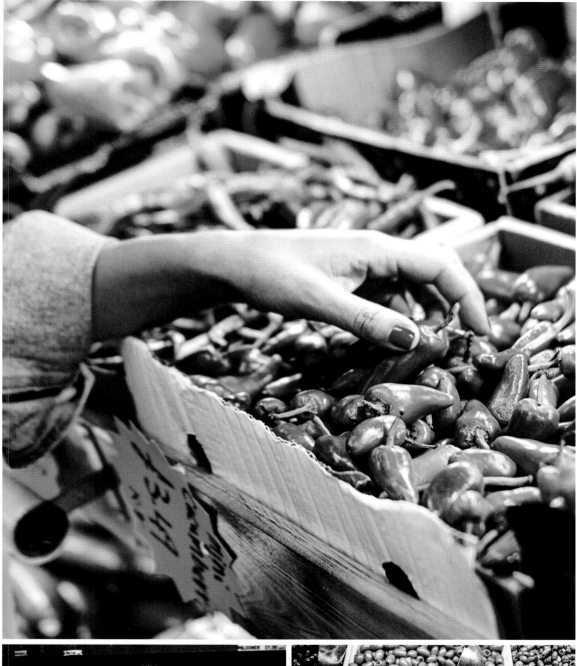

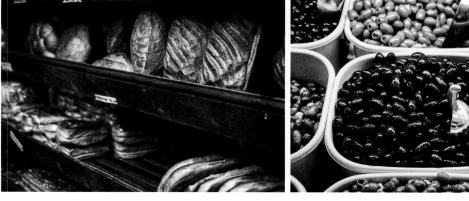

CRUNCHY ASIAN SALAD WITH GINGER DRESSING

Keep an eye on those tasty veggies. You want a reassuring crunch and a nicely toasted flavour to balance the tangy ginger dressing. Yummy.

SERVES 4   **DISH** LARGE ROASTING TRAY   **PREP** 20 MINS   **COOK** 8 MINS

250g tenderstem broccoli

150g fine green beans

2 tbsp sesame oil

¼ tsp chilli flakes, plus extra for topping

salt and pepper

100g cashews

2 carrots

150g radishes

1 beetroot

2 handfuls of mixed salad leaves

1 garlic clove

a thumb of fresh ginger (30g)

½ tbsp maple syrup

1 tbsp light soy sauce

extra virgin olive oil

1 tsp Dijon mustard

1 lemon

1 tbsp sesame seeds

Preheat the oven to 200°C fan/220°C/gas 7. Trim the ends off the broccoli, and top and tail the green beans. Put them both on a large roasting tray, drizzle with the sesame oil, then season with the chilli flakes and pinches of salt and pepper. Roast for 5 minutes, then sprinkle over the cashews and roast for another 3 minutes, until the nuts are golden and the veggies are starting to turn brown and are still slightly crunchy.

Meanwhile, chop the carrots into matchsticks (skins on) and thinly slice the radishes. Peel the beetroot and slice into matchsticks.

Remove the tray from the oven and add the carrot, beetroot and radishes, along with the mixed salad leaves. Peel and mince the garlic and ginger, and place in a small mixing bowl along with the maple syrup, soy sauce, 2 tablespoons of extra virgin olive oil, mustard and juice from the lemon. Stir until combined, then pour over the veggies and toss well. To finish, top the salad with extra chilli flakes (if you like it hot) and sesame seeds.

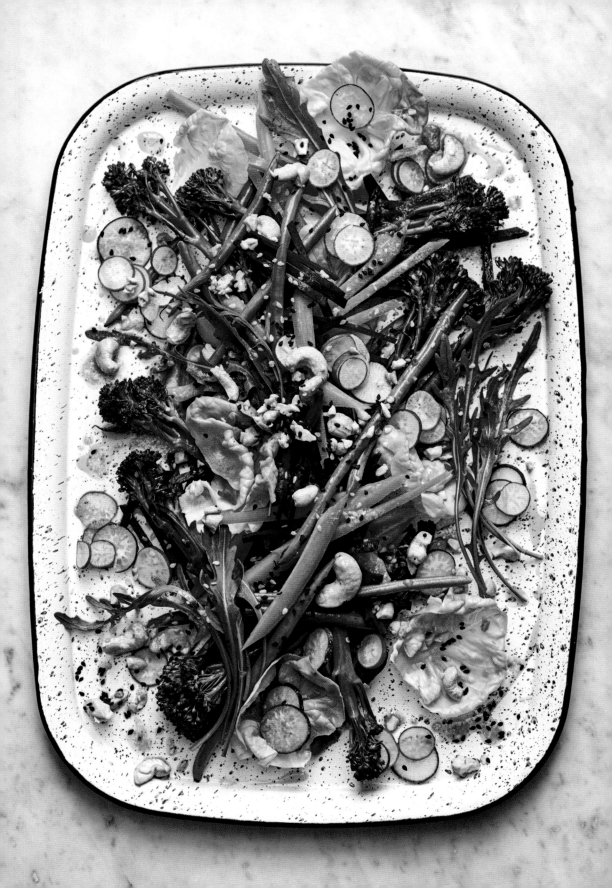

MINI GARDEN FLATBREADS

Can we all just take a second to appreciate za'atar? This miracle herb mix turns everything into Michelin-worthy grub, including these super easy homemade flatbreads.

SERVES 2   **DISH** LARGE BAKING TRAY   **PREP** 20 MINS   **COOK** 6–8 MINS

300g frozen peas

180g self-raising flour, plus extra for dusting

½ tsp baking powder

salt and pepper

130g vegan unsweetened yoghurt

2 tsp za'atar

olive oil

10 fresh mint leaves, plus extra for topping

1 lemon

40g jarred artichokes in oil, drained

2 radishes

salad cress, for topping

Preheat the oven to 230°C fan/250°C/gas 10. If your oven doesn't go this hot, get it as hot as you can. Put the frozen peas into a bowl and cover with hot water from a kettle, then leave to one side to thaw.

Put the flour, baking powder and a pinch of salt into a mixing bowl. Give the ingredients a stir, then mix in the vegan yoghurt. Dust a work surface with flour, then scoop out the dough and gently knead for a minute or so to form a ball. Slice the dough into 4 evenly sized pieces and roll out each piece into an oval flatbread shape about 13cm in length and roughly 2–3mm thick. Transfer the flatbreads to a large baking tray.

Mix the za'atar, 2 teaspoons of olive oil, and pinches of salt and pepper in a small bowl. Evenly drizzle the za'atar-infused oil over the flatbreads, using your fingers to spread it. Bake in the oven for 6–8 minutes, or until golden brown.

Drain the peas, then use a potato masher or a fork to roughly mash them until mostly broken down. Roughly chop the mint leaves and add them to the mashed peas, along with the juice from the lemon, and pinches of salt and pepper. Stir to combine, then, when the flatbreads are out of the oven, spoon the minty pea mixture over them.

Slice the artichokes into 1cm thick pieces and thinly slice the radishes. Top the flatbreads with the artichokes, radishes and salad cress, along with an extra pinch of pepper and half a dozen or so mint leaves. Yuuum.

> We use this quick flatbread recipe all the time to create mini pizza bases for an easy weeknight meal.

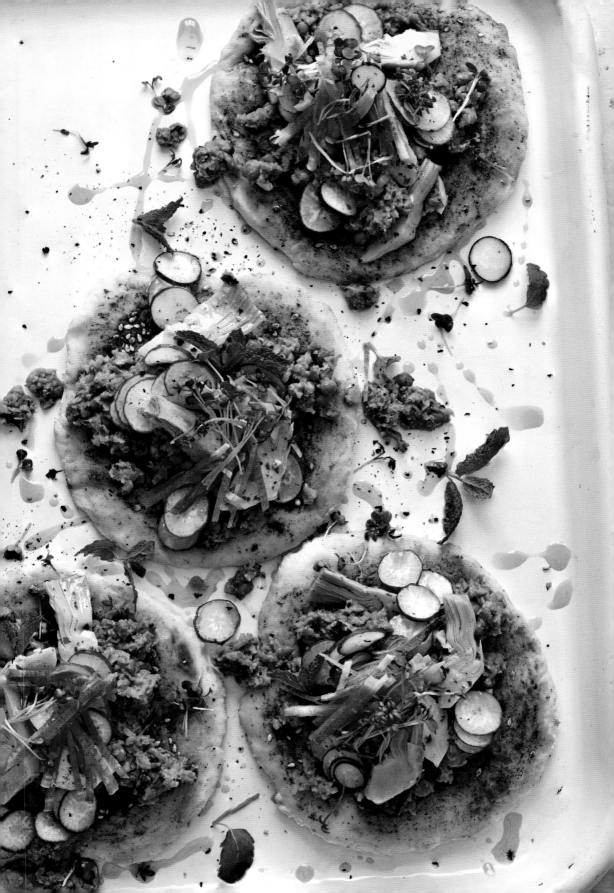

SWEET POTATO HASH WITH SCRAMBLED HARISSA TOFU

Brunch shouldn't be a chore and that's exactly where this harissa traybake comes in. Sweet potato brings added nutrition and the tofu proudly steps in as a sub for scrambled egg.

SERVES 4 **DISH** LARGE ROASTING TRAY **PREP** 15 MINS **COOK** 35 MINS

400g firm tofu

1 tsp turmeric

4 tsp rose harissa paste

salt

4 medium sweet potatoes (800g)

1 onion

4 tomatoes (350g)

olive oil

2 tsp paprika

2 green peppers

100g baby spinach

1 avocado

3 tbsp mixed seeds (pumpkin, sesame and sunflower)

Preheat the oven to 180°C fan/200°C/gas 6. Drain and press the tofu, if necessary. Using your hands, break the tofu into small pieces into a bowl. Add the turmeric, rose harissa paste and a large pinch of salt, then stir until the tofu is completely covered in the paste. Leave the tofu to marinate in the fridge while you complete the next steps.

Cut the sweet potatoes into 2cm pieces (we leave the skins on for extra nutrition), then transfer to a large roasting tray. Peel and thinly slice the onion, halve the tomatoes, then add both to the tray. Drizzle over 3 tablespoons of olive oil, sprinkle over the paprika and a large pinch of salt, then give everything a good mix. Roast in the oven for 20 minutes, stirring halfway through.

Meanwhile, slice the peppers into ½cm strips, discarding the seeds and stems. Add the peppers to the tray, give the veggies another stir, then scatter the tofu over the top. Return the tray to the oven for another 10 minutes.

Add the spinach leaves to the tray, then return it to the oven for 5 minutes. Meanwhile, slice the avocado in half, remove the stone, scoop out the flesh and slice each half. When the hash is ready, push the wilted spinach into the veggies, then place the sliced avocado on top and scatter over the mixed seeds to serve.

BALSAMIC BRUSSELS SPROUT SALAD

Welcome to the Brussels Sprouts Appreciation Society, where these mini cabbages are the stars of the show alongside sweet grapes and a balsamic Dijon dressing.

SERVES 4   **DISH** LARGE ROASTING TRAY   **PREP** 25 MINS   **COOK** 20 MINS

500g Brussels
sprouts

salt and pepper

olive oil

180g red seedless
grapes

¼ of a celeriac
(200g)

1 red onion

3 handfuls of baby
spinach

a handful of salted
peanuts

For the dressing:

2 tbsp balsamic
vinegar

1 tsp Dijon mustard

1 tsp maple syrup

3 tbsp extra virgin
olive oil

Preheat the oven to 200°C fan/220°C/gas 7. Trim the Brussels sprouts, remove any bad outer leaves, then cut in half and place on a large roasting tray. Sprinkle with salt and pepper and drizzle with 1 tablespoon of olive oil. Toss with your hands, then roast for 15 minutes.

Add the grapes to the tray and roast for 5 minutes more. Meanwhile, peel the celeriac and cut into matchsticks, and peel and slice the red onion.

Combine the dressing ingredients in a small mixing bowl with a pinch of salt and pepper.

Remove the tray from the oven, add the spinach leaves, celeriac, red onion and dressing, then toss with your hands. To finish, roughly chop the peanuts and sprinkle them all over the tray.

> Keen to avoid Brussels sprouts? You're probably not alone. Switch out for 1 large broccoli, broken down into bite-size florets.

NO-WASTE HARISSA CAULIFLOWER

Years ago we would have thrown the cauliflower stem and leaves in the bin. Nowadays they take centre stage and bring a new dimension to this one-tray wonder.

SERVES 4   **DISH** LARGE ROASTING TRAY   **PREP** 25 MINS   **COOK** 35 MINS

2 x 400g tins of chickpeas

salt and pepper

vegetable oil

2½ tbsp harissa paste

3 tbsp pomegranate molasses, plus extra for drizzling

1 medium cauliflower (700g)

1 medium broccoli (350g)

1 red onion

a handful of hazelnuts

a handful of fresh flat-leaf parsley (15g)

a handful of fresh mint (15g)

2 large handfuls of lamb's lettuce

For the dressing:

1 garlic clove

8 tbsp vegan plain yoghurt

1 lemon

Preheat the oven to 180°C fan/200°C/gas 6. Drain and rinse the chickpeas and put them into a large roasting tray. Season with salt and pepper, drizzle with 1 tablespoon of vegetable oil, then toss with your hands and roast for 15 minutes.

Meanwhile, combine the harissa paste, pomegranate molasses, 3 tablespoons of vegetable oil and a pinch of salt and pepper in a large mixing bowl. Next remove the leaves from the cauliflower (saving them for later) and cut the cauliflower and broccoli into bite-size florets and the stalks into 1cm cubes. Add to the bowl of harissa marinade and toss everything with your hands. Transfer to the tray and roast with the chickpeas for 10 minutes.

Roughly chop the cauliflower leaves, then remove the tray from the oven. Add the leaves to the tray and roast for 10 minutes.

Meanwhile, peel and slice the red onion, roughly chop the hazelnuts and pick the leaves off the parsley and mint. For the dressing, peel and chop the garlic, put it into a small bowl along with the vegan yoghurt, juice from the lemon and pinches of salt and pepper, and stir to combine.

Remove the tray from the oven and sprinkle with extra pinches of salt and pepper. Add the lamb's lettuce, red onion, yoghurt dressing, a drizzle of pomegranate molasses, the hazelnuts, mint and parsley. Voilà!

> Struggling to find pomegranate molasses? Simply combine 3 tablespoons of balsamic vinegar with 1 tablespoon of maple syrup, and sub it directly in this recipe.

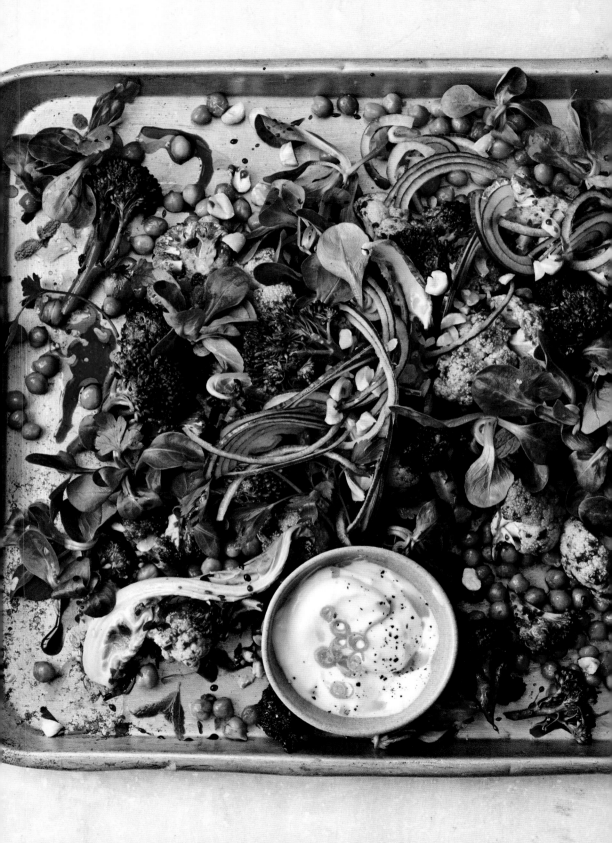

ROCKET HASSELBACK POTATOES

Perfectly crisp on the outside and soft in the middle, these hasselbacks are roasted with fresh rosemary and nestled among a vibrant mix of delicious morsels to create a stunning tray of food.

SERVES 4   **DISH** LARGE ROASTING TRAY   **PREP** 20 MINS   **COOK** 1 HR 15 MINS

4 sprigs of fresh rosemary

vegetable oil

salt and pepper

1 lemon

1.2kg medium potatoes

2 x 400g tin of cannellini beans

200g frozen peas

100g pistachios in shells

80g rocket

extra virgin olive oil

1 tsp Dijon mustard

50g radicchio

Preheat the oven to 180°C fan/200°C/gas 6. Pick the leaves from the rosemary sprigs, finely chop them and put them into a small bowl. Add 3 tablespoons of vegetable oil, ½ teaspoon of salt, ½ teaspoon of pepper and the zest from the lemon, and stir to combine. Leave to one side.

Place a potato between the handles of two wooden spoons and slice down into the potato (this will prevent the knife going all the way through) all the way along at 3mm intervals. Repeat for the rest of the potatoes. Transfer them to a large roasting tray and brush the herby oil evenly over the potatoes, pushing the rosemary down into the gaps. Roast for 70 minutes, until dark golden brown, turning the tray around halfway through to make sure they roast evenly.

Drain and rinse the cannellini beans. When the potatoes are ready, add the beans and frozen peas to the tray. Return to the oven for 5 minutes.

Meanwhile, peel the pistachios and put roughly three-quarters of them into a food processor (see tip below if you don't have a food processor), along with roughly two-thirds of the rocket, the juice from the lemon, 2 tablespoons of extra virgin olive oil, the mustard, 3 tablespoons of water, and pinches of salt and pepper. Process the ingredients to form a rough paste, adding a splash of extra water if it's too thick.

When the veggies are ready, stir in the radicchio and remaining rocket. Roughly chop the remaining pistachios, scatter them over the top, then drizzle the rocket sauce over everything. Delicious and nutritious!

> Don't have a food processor? Finely chop the peeled pistachios and rocket and add to a bowl, along with the juice of the lemon, the extra virgin olive oil, mustard, water and pinches of salt and pepper. Stir until combined.

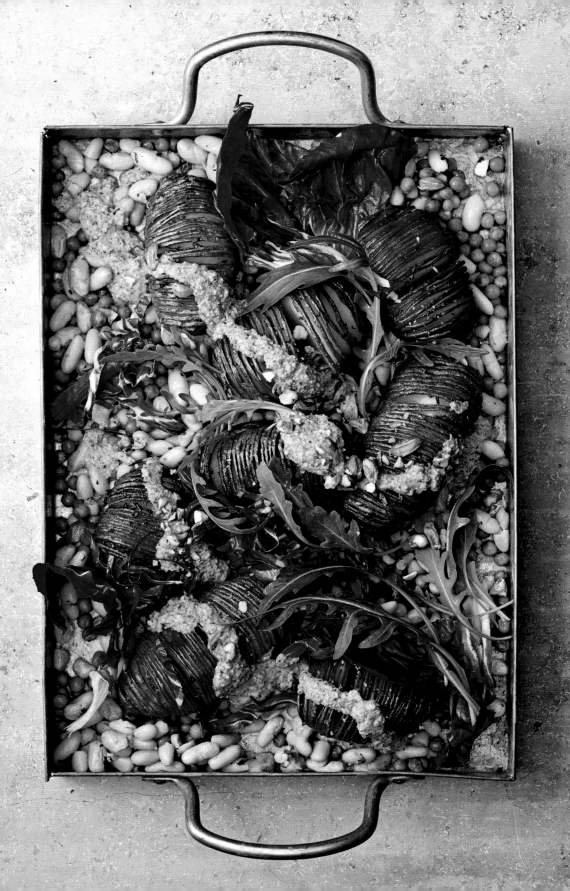

3 BEANS + CHICORY SALAD

We roast the slightly bitter chicory and combine it with a subtly sweet tahini dressing to create a healthy tray filled with mixed beans, fresh ginger and warm crusty bread.

SERVES 4   **DISH** LARGE ROASTING TRAY   **PREP** 10 MINS   **COOK** 20 MINS

250g fine green beans

1 x 400g tin of black beans

1 x 400g tin of pinto beans

4 heads of chicory

2 lemons

a thumb of fresh ginger (30g)

salt and pepper

olive oil

150g crusty bread (we use ciabatta)

4 tbsp tahini

1 tsp maple syrup

6 Brazil nuts

Preheat the oven to 200°C fan/220°C/gas 7.

Trim the ends off the green beans, drain and rinse the black and pinto beans, halve the chicory and slice one of the lemons. Transfer them all to a large roasting tray. Peel and chop the ginger, then add half to the tray and save the remainder for later. Sprinkle over large pinches of salt and pepper, and drizzle over 2 tablespoons of olive oil. Give everything a mix and roast for 15 minutes.

Tear the bread into big chunks and put them into a bowl, along with small pinches of salt and pepper and 1 tablespoon of olive oil. Give everything a good mix, then add the bread to the tray and return it to the oven for 5 minutes.

Meanwhile, combine the tahini in a bowl with the juice and zest of the remaining lemon, large pinches of salt and pepper, the remainder of the chopped ginger and 1 teaspoon of maple syrup. Stir in 4–5 tablespoons of water until it reaches a slightly runny consistency. Pour half the dressing over the veggies, then roughly slice the Brazil nuts and scatter them all over. Serve with the rest of the dressing alongside. Yum.

> We can't get enough of tahini, but occasionally we'll switch it for peanut butter or almond butter for a more nutty dressing.

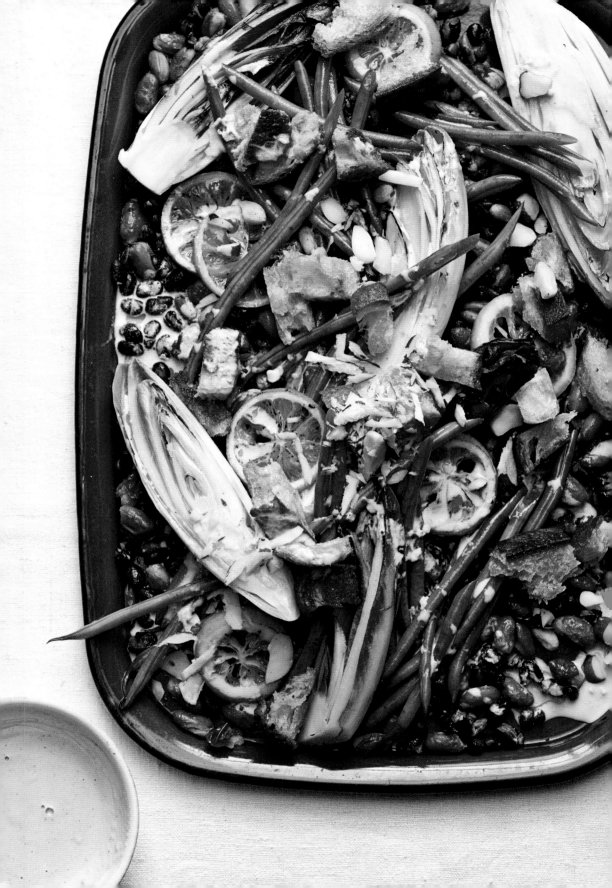

ROASTED VEGETABLE MEZZE

We love food that gets people talking around the dinner table, and this mezze is designed to do exactly that. Roasted za'atar veggies, couscous tabbouleh, yoghurt dip . . . take your pick.

SERVES 4–6 **DISH** LARGE ROASTING TRAY **PREP** 20 MINS **COOK** 40 MINS

2 medium beetroots (300g)

olive oil

50g couscous

2 medium courgettes (400g)

2 romano peppers

1½ tbsp za'atar, plus extra for sprinkling

salt and pepper

12 garlic cloves

a bunch of fresh flat-leaf parsley (30g)

a large handful of fresh mint (20g)

2 tomatoes

extra virgin olive oil

1½ lemons

200g vegan plain yoghurt

4 wholemeal pittas

200g crunchy veggies (we use yellow pepper and cucumber)

80g pitted green olives

Preheat the oven to 200°C fan/220°C/gas 7. Peel the beetroots and chop into 2cm pieces. Transfer to a large roasting tray and drizzle with 1 teaspoon of olive oil. Roast for 15 minutes.

Put the couscous into a mixing bowl and cover with 50ml of hot water from the kettle. Cover with a plate and leave to one side.

Slice the courgettes into batons and slice the peppers into 1cm strips. Add both to the tray and sprinkle over the za'atar, large pinches of salt and pepper and 2 teaspoons of olive oil. Give everything a mix and return the tray to the oven for 10 minutes. Add the garlic cloves (skins on) to the tray, give everything another mix and return it to the oven for another 10 minutes.

To create the tabbouleh, pick the parsley and mint leaves from their stalks, and roughly chop the leaves. Dice the tomatoes. As soon as the couscous is nice and fluffy, throw in the fresh herbs and tomatoes, along with 1 tablespoon of extra virgin olive oil, the juice from 1 lemon and pinches of salt and pepper. Stir to combine, then leave to one side.

Combine the yoghurt, the juice of the remaining lemon half and pinches of salt and pepper in a serving bowl. Leave to one side.

Slice the pittas into quarters and mix them into the roasted veggies to coat them in the herby oil. Return the tray to the oven again for 5 minutes. Then remove the garlic cloves from the tray and discard their skins. Chop 2 of the cloves and stir them into the tabbouleh, then chop the remaining 10 cloves and stir them into the yoghurt dip. Top the dip with a small pinch of za'atar.

Roughly chop the crunchy veggies and add them to the tray, along with the tabbouleh and olives. Serve alongside the garlic yoghurt dip.

> We're big fans of Middle Eastern spice blends. Baharat is another one of our favourites, and it could easily be switched in place for the za'atar.

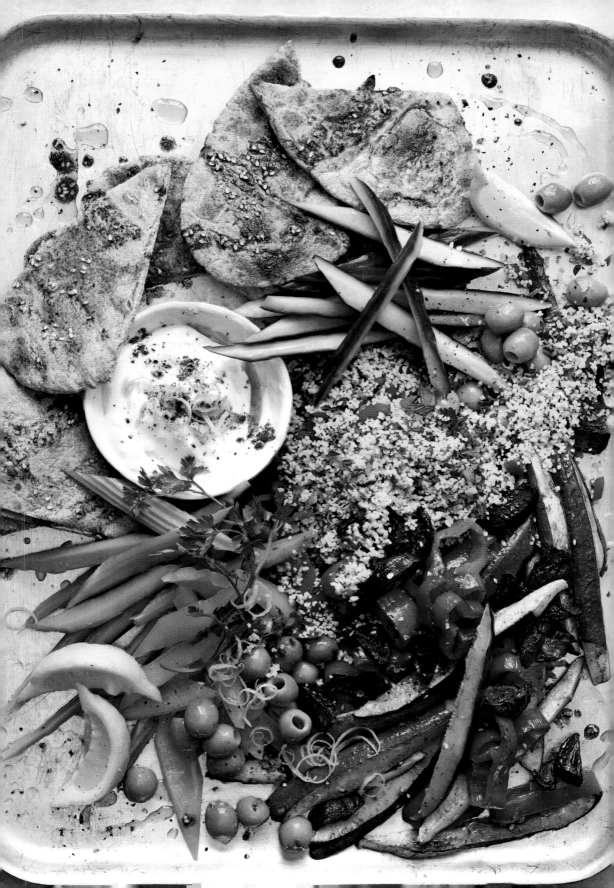

MEXICAN QUINOA SALAD

Light and fluffy quinoa, wonderfully warm spices and crunchy lettuce. This fuss-free salad is also great for meal prep if you're on the hunt for homemade lunch ideas.

SERVES 3–4   **DISH** CASSEROLE POT   **PREP** 20 MINS   **COOK** 30–35 MINS

1½ red onions

1 green chilli

olive oil

2 tsp ground cumin

1 tsp ground coriander

200g quinoa

1 x 400g tin of black beans

3 tomatoes (270g)

250ml vegetable stock

salt and pepper

1 gem lettuce

a large handful of fresh coriander (20g)

1 lime

vegan crème fraîche or vegan plain yoghurt, to serve

Peel and chop 1 red onion and thinly slice the green chilli. Put 2 tablespoons of olive oil into a casserole pot over a medium heat. As soon as the oil is hot, add the red onion, green chilli, cumin and ground coriander. Fry for 5 minutes.

Rinse the quinoa under cold water, then drain. Add it to the pot and fry for 2 minutes. Drain and rinse the black beans and roughly chop the tomatoes. Add them to the pot with the stock, ½ teaspoon of salt and a large pinch of pepper. Bring the quinoa to a boil, then lower the heat, cover, and simmer for 15–20 minutes, or until the liquid has been absorbed and the quinoa is light and fluffy. Remove the quinoa from the heat and leave the lid on for 5 minutes.

Meanwhile, chop the remaining red onion half and roughly chop the gem lettuce. Pick the coriander leaves off their stalks and roughly chop them. Stir them into the cooked quinoa, along with the juice of half the lime. Slice the remaining lime into wedges to serve, along with a few generous dollops of vegan crème fraîche or vegan plain yoghurt.

Throw in more fresh ingredients, such as avocado and mixed peppers, for added nutrition.

CAJUN MESS WITH CRUNCHY TORTILLA CRISPS

Invite your friends over. This easy Cajun mess is finger food at its finest and is best enjoyed in front of the TV with whatever tipple tickles your fancy.

SERVES 4 **DISH** LARGE ROASTING TRAY **PREP** 20 MINS **COOK** 25–30 MINS

3 mixed peppers (we use green, red and yellow)

1 red onion

5 tomatoes (450g)

2 x 400g tins of black beans

400g fresh corn kernels (or frozen sweetcorn)

3 tbsp Cajun seasoning

salt and pepper

olive oil

4 tortillas

To serve:

2 ripe avocados

extra virgin olive oil

1 lime

1 green chilli

a handful of fresh coriander (15g)

4 heaped tbsp vegan crème fraîche

Preheat the oven to 180°C fan/200°C/gas 6. Slice the peppers, peel and slice the red onion and dice the tomatoes. Drain and rinse the black beans, and put them on a roasting tray along with the prepared veggies, fresh corn kernels, Cajun seasoning, ½ teaspoon of salt, a large pinch of pepper and 2 tablespoons of olive oil. Toss to combine, then roast for 20 minutes, turning halfway.

Cut the tortillas into triangles and toss them in a bowl along with pinches of salt and pepper and 1 tablespoon of olive oil. Add them to the tray, then roast for 5–8 minutes, or until the tortilla chips are golden brown and crispy. Meanwhile, halve the avocados, remove the stones and spoon the flesh into a mixing bowl. Add 1 tablespoon of extra virgin olive oil, the juice of the lime, pinches of salt and pepper and 6–8 tablespoons of water. Mash the avocado dressing with a fork until fairly smooth and runny.

To serve, spoon over half the avocado sauce, then finely slice the green chilli and sprinkle it all over the tray. Pick the coriander leaves off their stalks and add them to the tray. Finish with a few spoonfuls of vegan crème fraîche and serve the rest of the sauce alongside.

Can't find vegan crème fraîche? Simply sub with vegan plain yoghurt.

FARRO, KALE + COCONUT SALAD

A sophisticated, warm and crispy kale salad, which uses the ancient grain farro and takes its inspiration from the beautiful island of Sri Lanka.

SERVES 4   **DISH** LARGE ROASTING TRAY   **PREP** 15 MINS   **COOK** 40 MINS

220g farro

80g cashews

4 handfuls of chopped kale

60g coconut flakes

olive oil

salt and pepper

½ a large cucumber (200g)

4 fresh figs

For the dressing:

2 green chillies

2 limes

extra virgin olive oil

2 tsp maple syrup

a small handful of fresh coriander (10g), plus extra for topping

Preheat the oven to 180°C fan/200°C/gas 6. Put the farro and 1 litre of hot water into a large roasting tray, then cover with baking paper or another large tray and bake for 35 minutes. Meanwhile, roughly chop the cashews.

Fluff the farro up with a fork, then add the kale, coconut flakes and cashews to the tray. Drizzle with 2 tablespoons of olive oil, season with salt and pepper and bake for 3–5 minutes, checking after 3 minutes to ensure the kale doesn't burn.

Meanwhile, thinly slice the cucumber and cut the figs in half. For the dressing, finely chop the green chillies, discarding the seeds, and put them into a small bowl along with the juice and zest of both the limes, 2 tablespoons of extra virgin olive oil, maple syrup and a pinch of salt. Pick the coriander leaves off their stalks, finely chop them and add them to the dressing. Stir to combine.

Remove the tray from the oven and top with the slices of cucumber and figs. Pour the dressing all over and toss. Scatter over the extra coriander leaves.

> Use up any leftover nuts you have in the cupboard. Walnuts, almonds and pecans can all be used to replace the cashews.

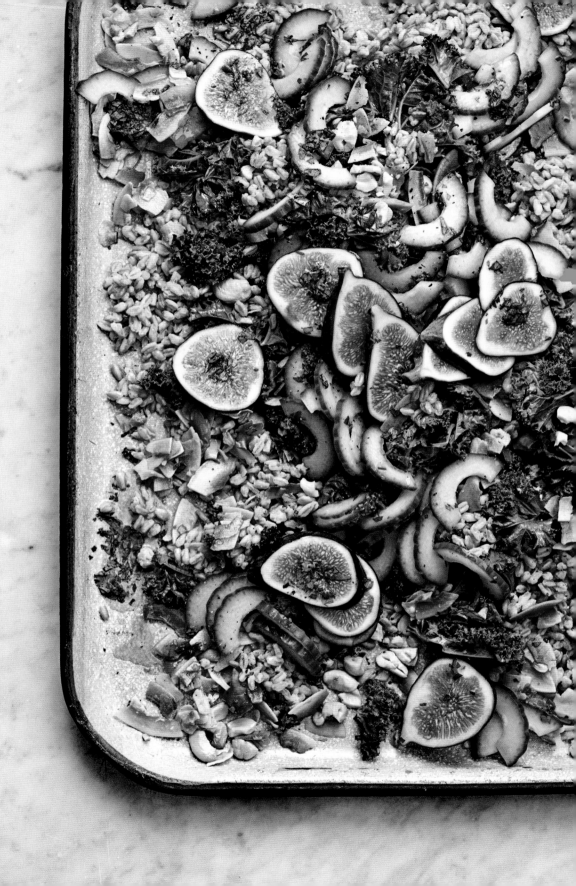

DINNERS

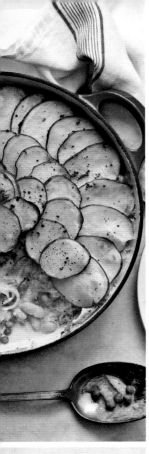

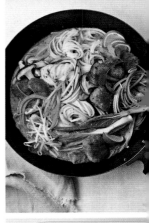

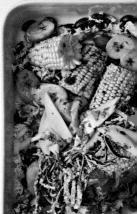

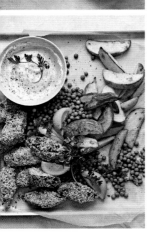

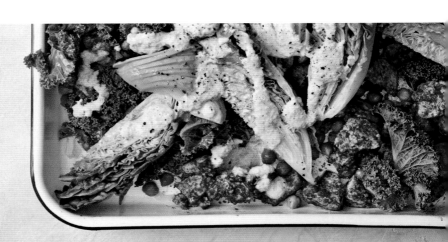

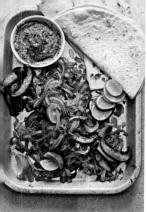
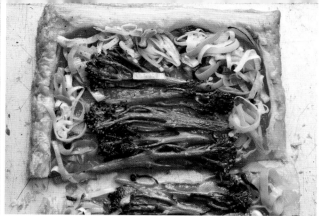

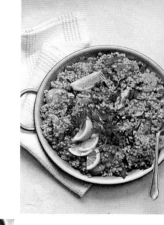

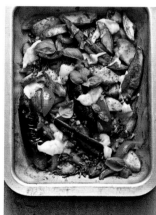

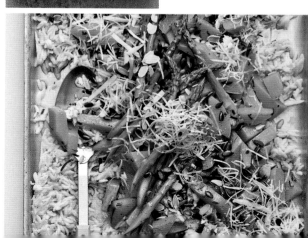

ROASTED POTATO ALLA NORMA

Our one-tray twist on the classic Sicilian pasta dish. We combine aubergines with roasted potatoes to create a big dinner with even bigger flavours.

SERVES 3–4   **DISH** LARGE ROASTING TRAY   **PREP** 15 MINS   **COOK** 1 HR

1kg Maris Piper potatoes

2 large aubergines (800g)

salt and pepper

olive oil

4 garlic cloves

4 tomatoes (350g)

1 x 400g tin of chopped tomatoes

1½ tbsp red wine vinegar

1½ tbsp capers

½ tsp dried oregano

½ tsp chilli flakes

80g vegan feta or mozzarella

a bunch of fresh basil (30g)

extra virgin olive oil

Preheat the oven to 180°C fan/200°C/gas 6. Cut the potatoes into quarters and transfer them to a large roasting tray.

Slice the aubergines into quarters lengthways, transfer to the tray and sprinkle over 1 teaspoon of salt, ½ teaspoon of pepper and drizzle over 3 tablespoons of olive oil. Toss with your hands, then roast in the oven for 35 minutes, turning halfway.

Peel and chop the garlic, then transfer to a medium mixing bowl. Quarter the tomatoes and add to the bowl along with the tinned tomatoes, vinegar, capers, dried oregano, chilli flakes, and a pinch of salt and pepper. Mix everything together.

Remove the tray from the oven and pour the tomato mixture all over, making sure it's evenly distributed. Push the aubergines down into the sauce a little to prevent them from catching, then return the tray to the oven for 20 minutes.

Slice the vegan cheese into small pieces. Remove the tray from the oven and sprinkle the vegan feta or mozzarella over the top, then pop the tray back into the oven for 3 minutes or until the cheese has melted into the sauce.

Meanwhile, roughly chop most of the basil leaves, leaving 4 or 5 whole to decorate. Remove the tray from the oven, stir in the chopped basil, then top with the reserved basil leaves. Drizzle over a splash of extra virgin olive oil and sprinkle over some freshly ground black pepper. Delicious!

> If you can't find a vegan version of feta or mozzarella, simply use your favourite vegan cheese.

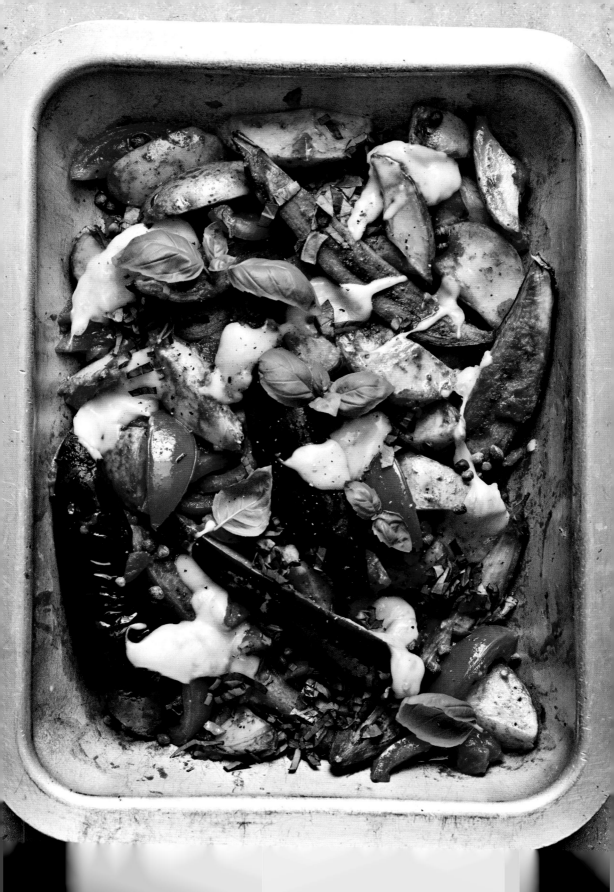

WEEKNIGHT PEANUT BUTTER UDON

Fuss-free cooking in 20 minutes? Yes please. Peanut butter is the hero in this recipe, helping to create a super flavoursome sauce with minimal effort.

SERVES 2 **DISH** WOK **PREP** 10 MINS **COOK** 10 MINS

1 onion

150g closed-cup
  mushrooms

2 garlic cloves

a thumb of fresh
  ginger (30g)

1 medium carrot

200g white cabbage

1 red pepper

vegetable oil

2 tbsp smooth
  peanut butter

2 tbsp dark soy
  sauce

1 tsp caster sugar

1 lime

2 tsp sesame oil

200g straight-to-wok
  udon noodles

3 spring onions

a handful of salted
  peanuts

1 tsp sesame seeds

chilli flakes, for
  topping

Start by prepping the veggies: peel and slice the onion, slice the mushrooms, peel and chop the garlic and ginger, slice the carrot into thin rounds at an angle (skin on), roughly chop the cabbage and cut the red pepper into 2½cm pieces.

Put a tablespoon of vegetable oil into a wok on a medium-high heat. Once hot, add the onion and fry for 2–3 minutes. Add the mushrooms, garlic, ginger, carrot, cabbage and red pepper and fry for 2–3 minutes more.

Meanwhile, in a small bowl, combine the peanut butter, soy sauce, sugar, the juice from half the lime and the sesame oil until smooth. Add the sauce to the wok along with the noodles and fry for 3 minutes.

Remove the wok from the heat. Chop the spring onions into 3cm pieces and toss them in. Roughly chop the peanuts and sprinkle them all over, along with the sesame seeds and as many chilli flakes as you like. Slice the remaining lime half into wedges to serve.

> Other light veggies like mangetout, green beans or baby corn will make a great addition to this dish. Add them along with the mushrooms.

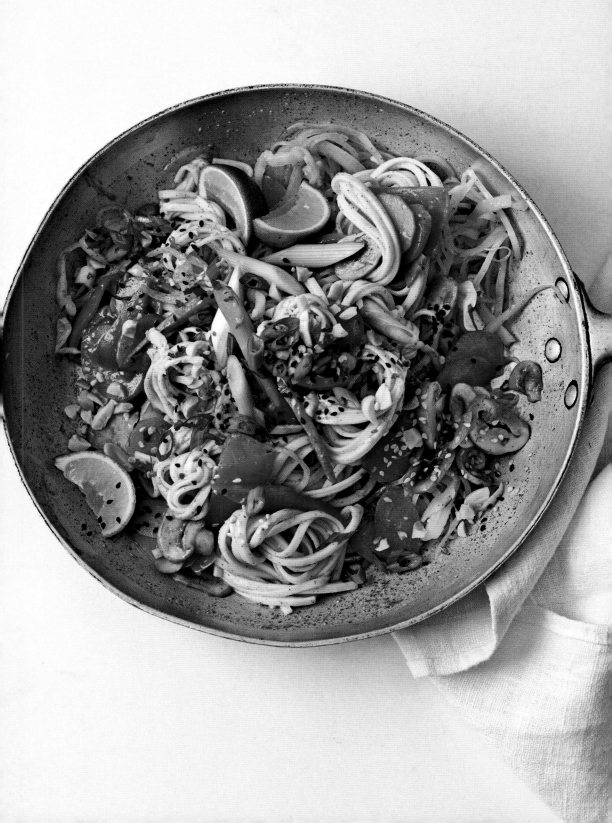

BROCCOLI, LEEK + CHUTNEY TART

This tart uses just a handful of ingredients to create a super-simple dinner. Expect sweet and tangy flavours, and satisfyingly crunchy tenderstem broccoli.

SERVES 4   **DISH** LARGE BAKING TRAY   **PREP** 15 MINS   **COOK** 30 MINS

320g pre-rolled vegan puff pastry

3 tbsp mango chutney

150g vegan cream cheese

4 sprigs of fresh thyme

1 leek

200g tenderstem broccoli

olive oil

salt and pepper

Preheat the oven to 180°C fan/200°C/gas 6.

Unroll the puff pastry on to a large baking tray, keeping it on the paper that it was rolled in. Use a knife to lightly score a 2cm border around the pastry, then spread the mango chutney evenly over the pastry, inside the border, followed by the vegan cream cheese. Pick the thyme leaves off their stalks and scatter them over the cream cheese.

Slice the leek and scatter it over the cream cheese, then add the tenderstem broccoli in single rows down the centre from top to bottom, aligned with the shorter edge. Drizzle over 1 tablespoon of olive oil and sprinkle large pinches of salt and pepper on top. Then brush the border of the pastry with olive oil. Bake in the oven for 30 minutes or until the pastry is golden brown.

> Any type of chutney will do well here. Try caramelized onion chutney or tomato chutney to capture a similar sweet flavour.

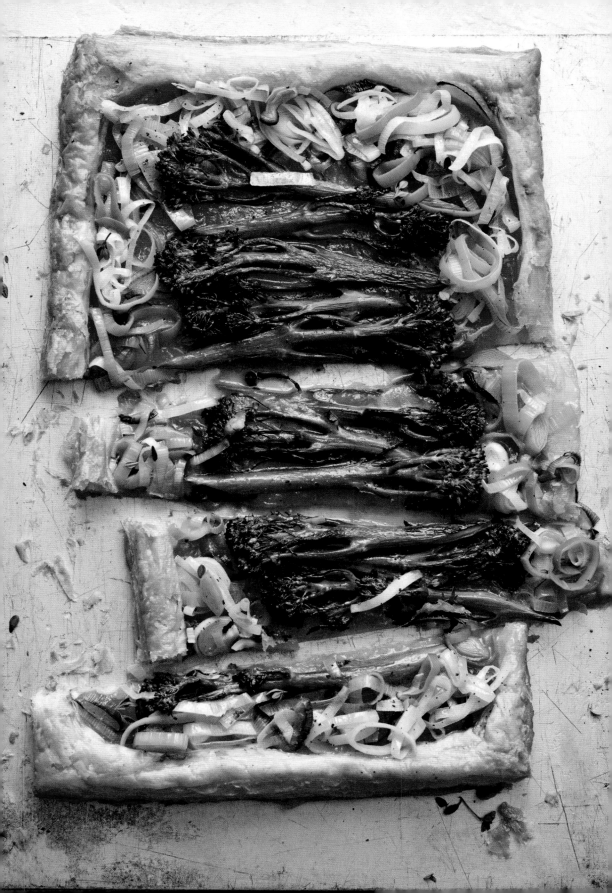

PEARL BARLEY CHILLI

Pearl barley is a super substitute for rice. It's nutritionally dense and we simply add it to the pot to keep things easy. Dial the heat up or down to your liking.

SERVES 4   **DISH** CASSEROLE POT   **PREP** 15 MINS   **COOK** 55–65 MINS

1 red onion

4 garlic cloves

2 red chillies

olive oil

½ tsp chilli flakes, plus extra for topping

1 tbsp smoked paprika

2 tsp ground cumin

1 tsp ground cinnamon

200g pearl barley

2 x 400g tinned beans (we use kidney and black)

500ml vegetable stock

2 x 400g tins of plum tomatoes

4 tbsp tomato purée

salt

30g dark chocolate

a handful of fresh coriander (15g)

vegan plain yoghurt

crusty bread, to serve

Peel and chop the onion and garlic, and dice one of the chillies (discard the seeds if you prefer a less spicy chilli). Heat 1 tablespoon of olive oil in a casserole pot over a medium heat. As soon as the oil is hot, add the onion, garlic and chilli and fry for 10 minutes, stirring occasionally until the onion is soft and lightly browned.

Next add the chilli flakes, smoked paprika, cumin and cinnamon. Reduce to a low-medium heat and cook the spices for 2 minutes.

Rinse the pearl barley in cold water, then add to the pot and toast for 3 minutes, stirring a few times.

Drain and rinse the beans, and add them to the pot along with the vegetable stock and tinned tomatoes. Pour 100ml of hot water from a kettle into each of the empty tomato tins (200ml in total), swirl them around to catch the remaining juice, and pour it into the pot, followed by the tomato purée and a large pinch of salt. Stir to combine, bring the chilli to the boil, then lower the heat and simmer for 40–50 minutes, or until the barley is cooked but still has a bite.

When the chilli is ready, roughly chop the dark chocolate and stir it into the pot. Cook for another 2 minutes, season to taste with salt, if necessary, then remove from the heat.

Thinly slice the remaining red chilli and pick the coriander leaves off their stalks. Top the chilli with a generous drizzle of vegan yoghurt, the coriander leaves, the sliced chilli and a sprinkle of chilli flakes, and serve with slices of crusty bread.

> Fry some chopped courgettes and peppers along with the onion for extra nutrition.

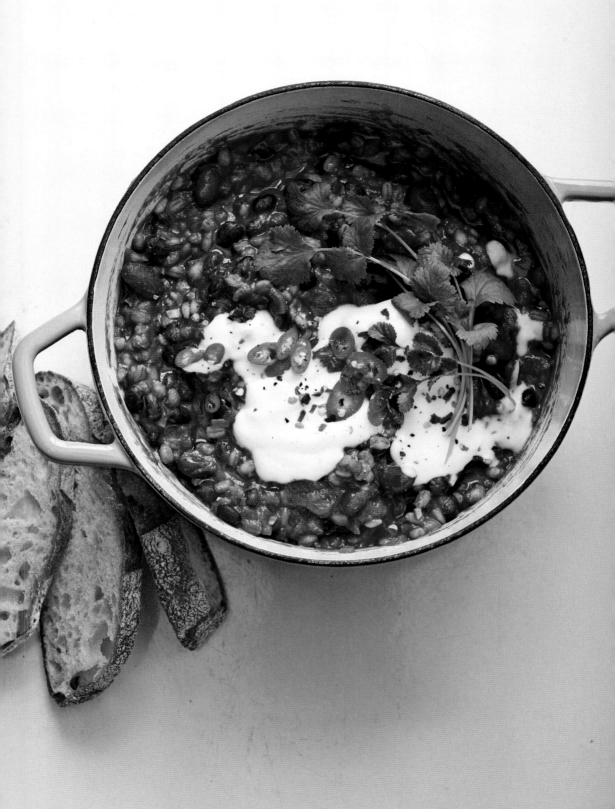

MUSHROOM TIKKA MASALA

We're completely obsessed with curry. We're almost always combining different spices to discover new blends, and this tikka masala is without doubt one of our favourite creations.

SERVES 4   **DISH** CASSEROLE POT   **PREP** 20 MINS   **COOK** 35 MINS

2–3 tbsp vegan margarine

1 onion

500g chestnut mushrooms

4 garlic cloves

½ a thumb of fresh ginger (15g)

3 cardamom pods

½ tsp turmeric

2 tsp ground cumin

1 tsp garam masala

1 tsp ground coriander

¼ tsp chilli powder

1 tsp smoked paprika

¼ tsp ground cinnamon

400g fresh tomatoes

3 tbsp tomato purée

½ tsp sugar

2 green chillies

100ml single soya cream

salt and pepper

a handful of fresh coriander (15g)

4 vegan naans

Put 2 tablespoons of margarine into a casserole pot on a medium-high heat. While the pot heats up, peel and slice the onion, then add it to the pot and fry for 8 minutes, or until golden.

Remove any large stalks from the mushrooms and finely chop the stalks. Then add the whole mushrooms and the chopped stalks to the pot, and fry for 8 minutes. Add an extra tablespoon of margarine here, if needed.

Meanwhile, peel and finely grate the garlic and ginger. Crush the cardamom pods in a pestle and mortar, remove the outer husks and grind the seeds. Then add the garlic, ginger, cardamom seeds and all the remaining spices to the pot. Fry for 3 minutes.

Dice the tomatoes and add them to the pot along with the tomato purée and sugar, and fry for 3 minutes.

Halve the green chillies lengthways and add them to the pot along with 150ml of hot water, the single soya cream, ½ teaspoon of salt and a generous pinch of pepper. Simmer for 10 minutes, stirring occasionally.

Pick the coriander leaves off their stalks and sprinkle them over the top, then toast the naans to serve.

Perfect for making in big batches and freezing, for a day when you just want to put your feet up in front of the TV.

WILD MUSHROOM + ASPARAGUS RISOTTO

Soy sauce is a staple in vegan cooking. Here it adds depth and a much-needed savouriness, enhancing the 'mushroomy' flavour in this classic risotto.

SERVES 4 **DISH** SHALLOW CASSEROLE PAN **PREP** 15 MINS **COOK** 40–50 MINS

200g wild mushrooms (we use chanterelles)

12 asparagus spears (300g)

1 onion

2 garlic cloves

a bunch of fresh flat-leaf parsley (30g)

olive oil

salt and pepper

3 vegetable stock cubes

350g Arborio rice

250ml dry white wine

½ a lemon

1 tsp light soy sauce

50g vegan Parmesan

Slice the mushrooms in half. Trim the tough ends off the asparagus, cut in half lengthways and slice into 4–5cm pieces. Peel and chop the onion and garlic, and pick the parsley leaves off their stalks. Roughly chop most of the leaves, reserving a small handful for topping, and finely chop the stalks.

Put 1 tablespoon of olive oil in a shallow casserole pan over a medium-high heat. As soon as the oil is hot, add the mushrooms with a pinch of salt and pepper and fry for 2 minutes. Add the asparagus and fry for 3 minutes.

Remove from the heat, then transfer the mushrooms and asparagus, including any juices, to a bowl. Wipe the pan clean, then return it to a low-medium heat and add 1 tablespoon of olive oil. As soon as the oil is hot, add the onion to the pan and fry for 5–10 minutes, until softened. Add the garlic and parsley stalks to the pan and fry for 2 minutes.

Meanwhile, put the kettle on to boil and put 1 stock cube into a measuring jug, ready for later. It's important to prepare the stock in batches so it remains hot.

Add the rice to the pan and fry for 3–4 minutes to 'toast' the grains, stirring occasionally. Once the rice is translucent at the edges, turn the heat up to medium-high, pour in the wine and cook until it has evaporated.

Pour 500ml of hot water from the kettle into the jug containing the stock cube. Stir until it has dissolved, then add the stock to the pan roughly 150ml at a time, stirring regularly to prevent the rice sticking to the bottom of the pan. As soon as your batch of stock is about to run out, get the kettle on the boil again and prepare the next 500ml of stock. Keep the rice cooking over a medium-high heat, adding more stock as you go, and it should take approximately 18–20 minutes until it's al dente.

When the rice is almost ready, add a large pinch of pepper, the juice from the lemon half, soy sauce and chopped parsley leaves. Grate in most of the vegan Parmesan and give it a good stir. The stock, soy sauce and vegan Parmesan should bring enough salt to the dish, but trust your palate and season to taste. Cook the risotto for another minute, then stir in the asparagus and mushrooms, including any juices. If the rice has begun to thicken up, simply add a splash of any remaining stock or hot water, and stir through.

To serve, grate the remaining vegan Parmesan over the top and sprinkle over the rest of the parsley leaves and a pinch of freshly ground black pepper. Delicious.

Instead of vegan Parmesan, try adding 6 tablespoons of nutritional yeast and an extra pinch of salt for a similar tangy and cheesy flavour.

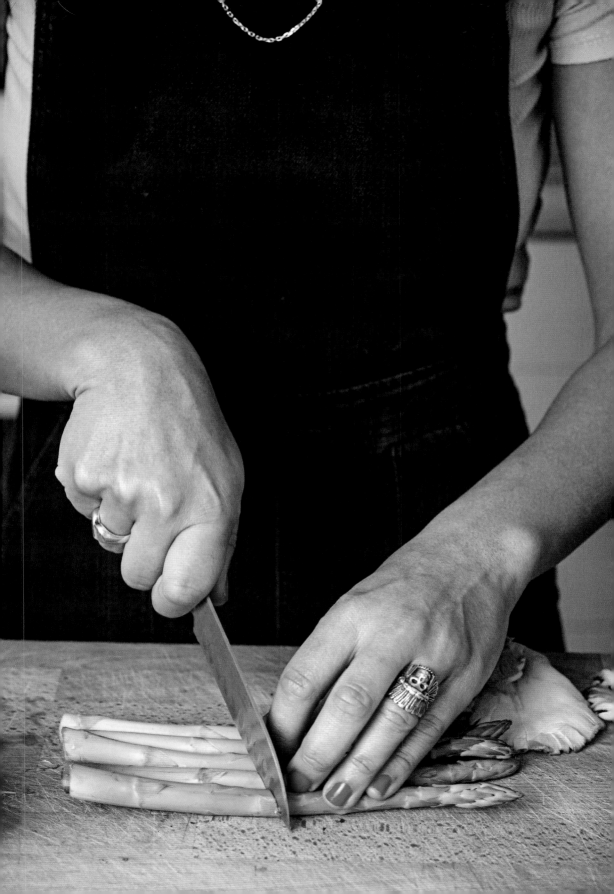

SHIITAKE LAKSA

This South East Asian-inspired soup uses fresh ingredients to deliver bags of flavour. Kaffir lime leaves and lemongrass are both game changers, and you'll now find them in most big supermarkets.

SERVES 2   **DISH** WOK   **PREP** 20 MINS   **COOK** 40 MINS

2 shallots

a thumb of fresh ginger (30g)

3 garlic cloves

2 red chillies

4 kaffir lime leaves

1 tsp ground turmeric

1 tbsp light soy sauce

a handful of fresh coriander (15g), plus extra for serving

1 lemongrass stalk

vegetable oil

125g shiitake mushrooms

500ml vegetable stock

50g rice noodles

1 small carrot

½ a courgette

2 baby pak choi

½ a 400g tin of light coconut milk

a handful of beansprouts

8 tofu puffs

1 lime

Peel and roughly chop the shallots, then peel the ginger and garlic. Put them in a food processor (see tip below if you don't have a food processor) along with 1 red chilli, the kaffir lime leaves, turmeric, soy sauce and coriander, including the stalks. Remove and discard the tough outer layer of the lemongrass, then chop the softer inner layers and add to the food processor. Blitz this curry paste until mostly broken down, scraping down the sides as you go, if necessary.

Heat 1 tablespoon of vegetable oil in a wok on a medium-high heat. While the oil heats up, slice the mushrooms, then add them to the wok and fry for 3–5 minutes until browned. Transfer the mushrooms to a bowl. Add 1 tablespoon of vegetable oil to the wok, reduce the heat and fry the curry paste for 15 minutes.

Add the vegetable stock along with 100ml of hot water from the kettle, and simmer gently for 5 minutes. Then add the noodles and cook for a further 5 minutes, or until the noodles are ready.

Meanwhile, peel the carrot and courgette into ribbons, then cut each ribbon in half lengthways. Cut the pak choi in half lengthways. Add the veggies to the wok along with the coconut milk and leave to simmer for a few minutes, until the pak choi has slightly softened.

Remove the wok from the heat and stir in the mushrooms, beansprouts and tofu puffs so they heat through. To finish, sprinkle over some coriander leaves and serve with wedges of lime.

> Don't have a food processor? Finely chop the shallots, ginger, garlic, chilli, kaffir lime leaves and lemongrass, and add them to a pestle and mortar. Once mostly broken down, add the turmeric, soy sauce and coriander, and grind into a paste.

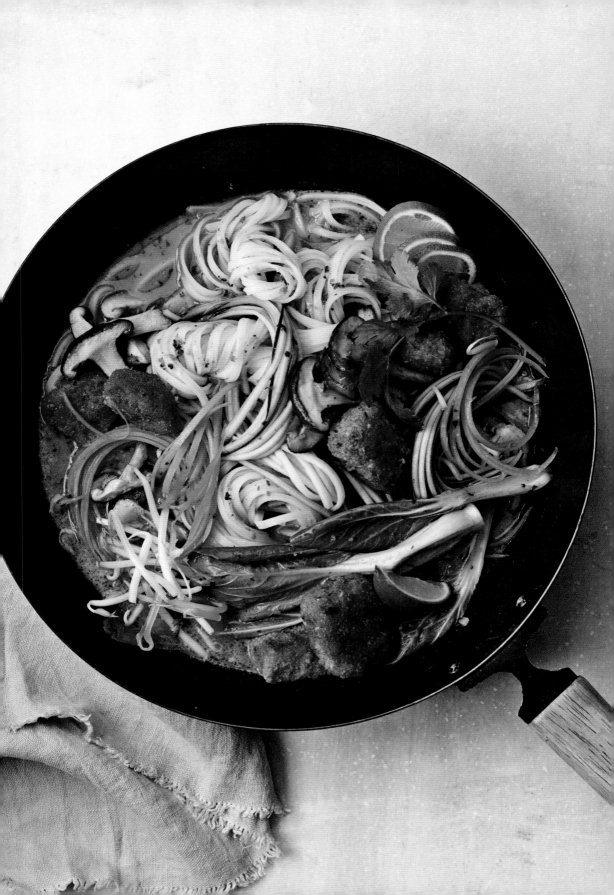

SEASIDE TOFISH GOUJONS + CHIPS

Vegan fish. Homemade tartare sauce. Crispy wedges. There's a lot to love about this simple seaside-inspired feast.

SERVES 4   **DISH** LARGE ROASTING TRAY   **PREP** 30 MINS   **COOK** 40 MINS

400g firm tofu

4 Maris Piper potatoes (850g)

salt and pepper

olive oil

2 lemons

1 large sheet of nori

60ml unsweetened plant-based milk

1 tbsp apple cider vinegar

2 tsp Cajun seasoning, plus 2 tbsp

80g panko breadcrumbs

1½ tsp garlic powder

¾ tsp onion powder

1½ tbsp dried dill

300g frozen peas

For the tartare sauce:

1 tbsp capers

1 gherkin

a handful of fresh flat-leaf parsley (15g)

125g vegan mayonnaise

Preheat the oven to 220°C fan/240°C/gas 9 and line a large roasting tray with baking paper. Drain and press the tofu, if necessary.

Slice the potatoes into wedges, then spread them out on the baking tray, season with salt and pepper and add a drizzle of olive oil. Toss with your hands, then bake for 20 minutes.

Cut the tofu into 12 strips about 2cm wide. Season with salt and pepper and squeeze over the juice of half a lemon. Cut the nori into 12 strips similar in size to the tofu strips. Line one side of each piece of tofu with a strip of nori.

In a small bowl, combine the milk with the vinegar and 2 teaspoons of Cajun seasoning. In a separate bowl, combine the breadcrumbs with the garlic powder, onion powder, dill, 2 tablespoons of Cajun seasoning, a pinch of salt and pepper and 2 tablespoons of olive oil. Holding the nori in place, dip each strip of tofu first in the wet mixture then in the dry mixture.

Remove the baking tray from the oven. Push the chips up to one end and put the tofu strips at the other end in a single layer. Bake everything for 10 minutes. Remove the baking tray from the oven and clear a space for the peas, then add them to the tray and bake for another 8–10 minutes, until everything is golden brown and the peas are soft.

Meanwhile, prepare the tartare sauce. Finely chop the capers, gherkin and parsley leaves (leaving some parsley to garnish with later). Throw them into a small bowl along with the vegan mayonnaise and give everything a good stir.

Cut the remaining lemon into wedges. Once the goujons and chips have finished cooking, squeeze the juice from a couple of the wedges all over and decorate with the remaining wedges. Finish with the remaining chopped parsley and a sprinkling of salt.

> Some brands of tofu will require pressing underneath a heavy object or squeezing between your hands to remove excess moisture.

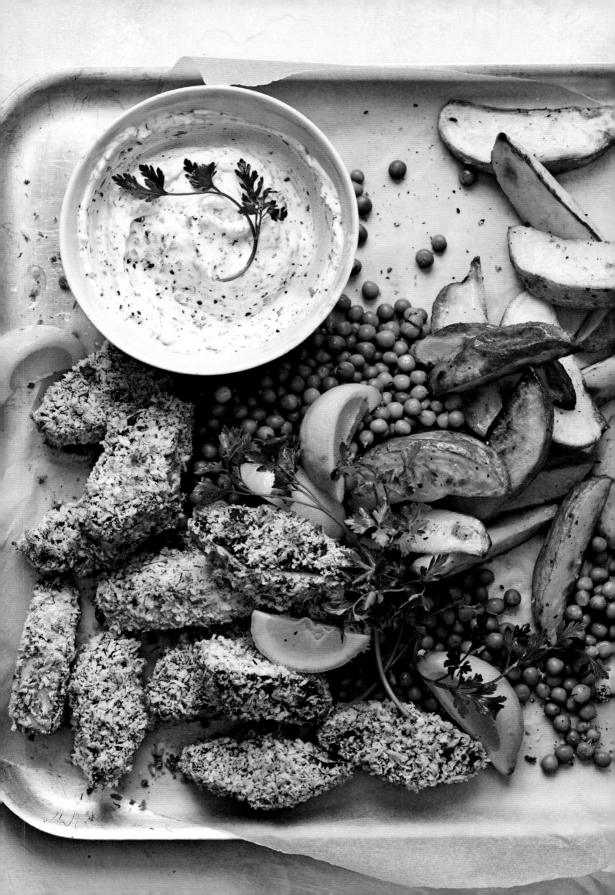

CREAMY CAULIFLOWER KORMA

Ben used to have a personal vendetta against korma. Apparently it was always the safe and boring option at a curry house. But our vegan version has renewed his faith in this classic creamy curry.

SERVES 4   **DISH** CASSEROLE POT   **PREP** 20 MINS   **COOK** 30 MINS

vegetable oil

1 onion

3 medium sweet
    potatoes (450g)

½ a large cauliflower
    (400g)

4 garlic cloves

a thumb of fresh
    ginger (30g)

2 tsp ground turmeric

1½ tbsp garam
    masala

½ tsp ground nutmeg

250ml vegan single
    cream

400ml vegetable
    stock

80g ground almonds

1 tbsp maple syrup

salt and pepper

To serve (optional):

a small handful of
    fresh coriander
    (10g)

a handful of raisins

a handful of toasted
    almond flakes

4 vegan naans

Put 2 tablespoons of vegetable oil into a casserole pot on a medium heat. While the oil heats up, peel and dice the onion, then add it to the pot and fry for 5 minutes until golden brown.

Peel the sweet potatoes and dice into 2½cm chunks, then add to the pot and fry for 10 minutes.

Trim the cauliflower into florets, and leave to one side. Peel and chop the garlic and ginger, then add to the pot along with the turmeric, garam masala and nutmeg. Fry for 2 minutes, adding an extra splash of oil, if needed.

Add the cauliflower florets to the pot along with 200ml of vegan single cream, the vegetable stock, ground almonds, maple syrup and a large pinch of salt and pepper. Bring to the boil, then reduce the heat and simmer with the lid on for 10 minutes, or until the cauliflower is soft. If the sauce is a little thin, simmer for an extra 5 minutes with the lid off.

Remove the korma from the heat. Pick the coriander leaves off their stalks. Stir in the raisins, and top with a swirl of the remaining cream, the coriander leaves and almond flakes. Finally, heat the naans in a toaster or microwave and serve.

> If you have any carrots, broccoli or mushrooms lying around, add them along with the sweet potato – they'll be a welcome addition.

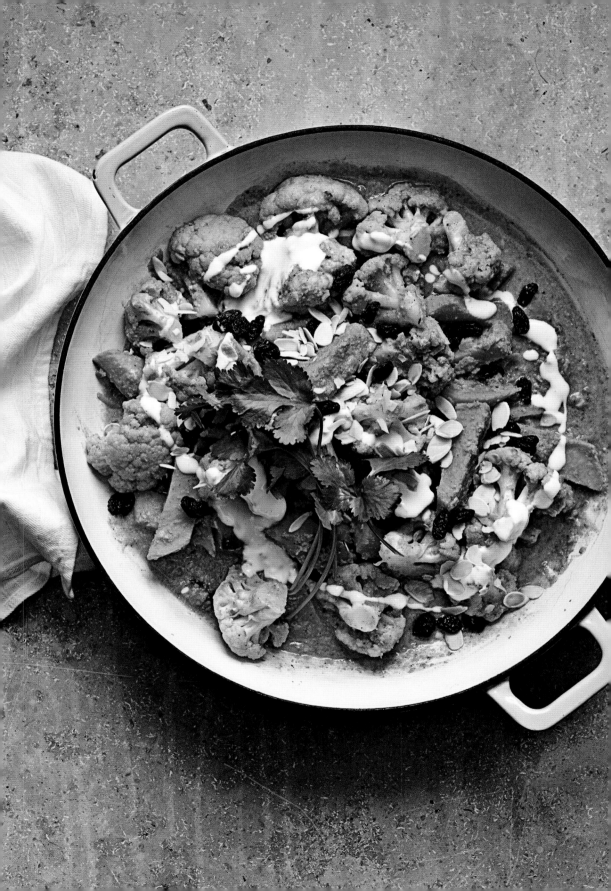

ALOO GOBI TRAYBAKE

A true staple. Aloo gobi makes a regular appearance when we order our favourite Indian takeaway. So we decided to reinvent the dish and give it the one-tray treatment.

SERVES 4 **DISH** LARGE ROASTING TRAY **PREP** 25 MINS **COOK** 55 MINS

1kg Maris Piper potatoes

1 large cauliflower (1kg)

vegetable oil

1½ tbsp ground cumin, plus 1 tsp

1 tbsp ground coriander, plus 1 tsp

2 tsp ground turmeric, plus ½ tsp

2 tsp nigella seeds

½ tbsp garam masala, plus ½ tsp

salt and pepper

a large thumb of fresh ginger (30g)

4 garlic cloves

2 tbsp tomato purée

500ml vegetable stock

300g cherry tomatoes

½ tsp chilli flakes

1 lime

1 onion

a handful of coconut flakes

1 red chilli

a handful of fresh coriander (15g)

Preheat the oven to 200°C fan/220°C/gas 7. Cut the larger potatoes in half and trim the cauliflower into florets (save the leaves for later). Add the potatoes and florets to a large mixing bowl along with 4 tablespoons of vegetable oil, 1½ tablespoons of cumin, 1 tablespoon of coriander, 2 teaspoons of turmeric, 2 teaspoons of nigella seeds, ½ tablespoon of garam masala and generous pinches of salt and pepper. Gently toss with your hands until evenly coated, then pick out the potato and place it on a roasting tray. Roast for 30 minutes.

To make the sauce, peel and chop the ginger and garlic and put both into a mixing bowl with the tomato purée, stock, chilli flakes, the juice of half the lime and the rest of the spices (1 teaspoon of cumin, 1 teaspoon of ground coriander, ½ teaspoon of turmeric, and ½ teaspoon of garam masala). Stir to combine and set to one side.

Take the tray out of the oven and scatter the cauliflower florets and cherry tomatoes on top, then pour the sauce all over. Peel and quarter the onion and add it to the tray, along with the cauliflower leaves from earlier. Bake for 20 minutes, then scatter over the coconut flakes and roast for another 5 minutes.

Cut the remaining lime half into wedges and spread over the tray. Slice the chilli, roughly chop the leaves from the coriander, and sprinkle both over the aloo gobi.

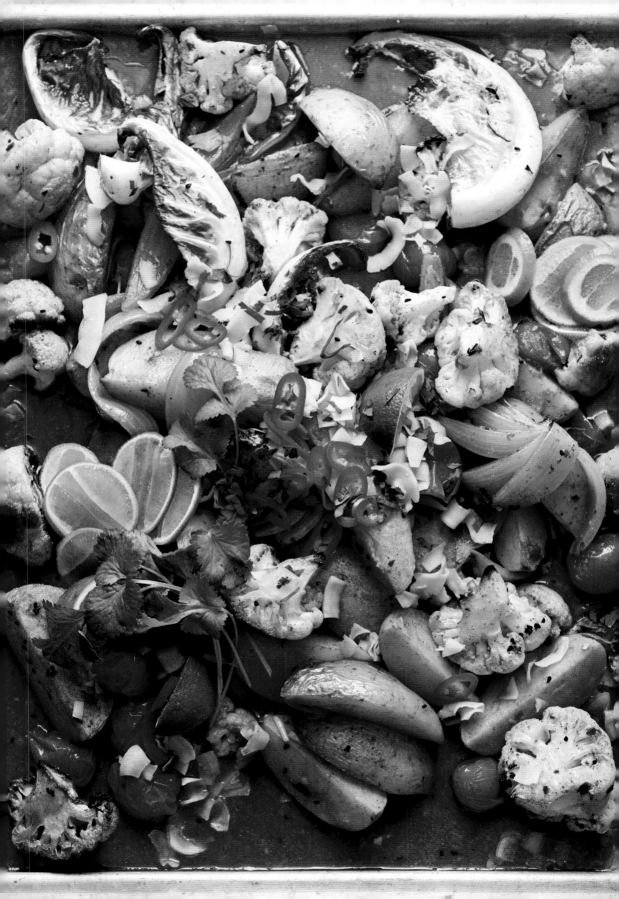

SUPER GREEN GNOCCHI

Some days the last thing we want to do is spend our entire evening in the kitchen. That's where our super green gnocchi steps in. Flavoursome and fuss-free, just how we like it.

SERVES 4 **DISH** LARGE SAUCEPAN **PREP** 10 MINS **COOK** 4–6 MINS

150g green beans

12 asparagus spears (300g)

800g vegan gnocchi

1 small garlic clove

a bunch of fresh basil (30g), plus extra for serving

150g baby spinach

40g walnuts

extra virgin olive oil

3 tbsp nutritional yeast

½ a lemon

salt and pepper

Bring a large saucepan of salted water to the boil over a high heat. Meanwhile, trim the ends off the beans. Trim the tough ends off the asparagus and slice into thirds. Add both to the boiling water and simmer for 3–4 minutes, then use a slotted spoon to transfer the veggies to a large bowl.

Bring the water back to a fast boil, and carefully add the gnocchi. Cook for 1–2 minutes, until they float to the surface, then use a slotted spoon to transfer them to the bowl of veggies, reserving the cooking water.

Peel the garlic, pick the leaves off the basil and add both to a food processor (see tip below if you don't have a food processor) along with the spinach, walnuts, 2 tablespoons of extra virgin olive oil, the nutritional yeast, the juice from the lemon half, and a pinch of salt and pepper. Add 2 tablespoons of the reserved cooking water and blend until you have a smooth pesto. Season to taste with extra salt and pepper, if necessary.

Discard the rest of the cooking water, then put the gnocchi and veggies back into the pan. Add every drop of the delicious pesto and stir to combine, until the gnocchi and veggies are completely covered. Finish with an extra pinch of pepper and top with a few fresh basil leaves. Yum!

> Don't have a food processor? Simply finely chop the garlic, spinach and basil, then add the walnuts and nutritional yeast and continue chopping until fine. Transfer to a bowl and add the oil, lemon juice, reserved water and salt and pepper.

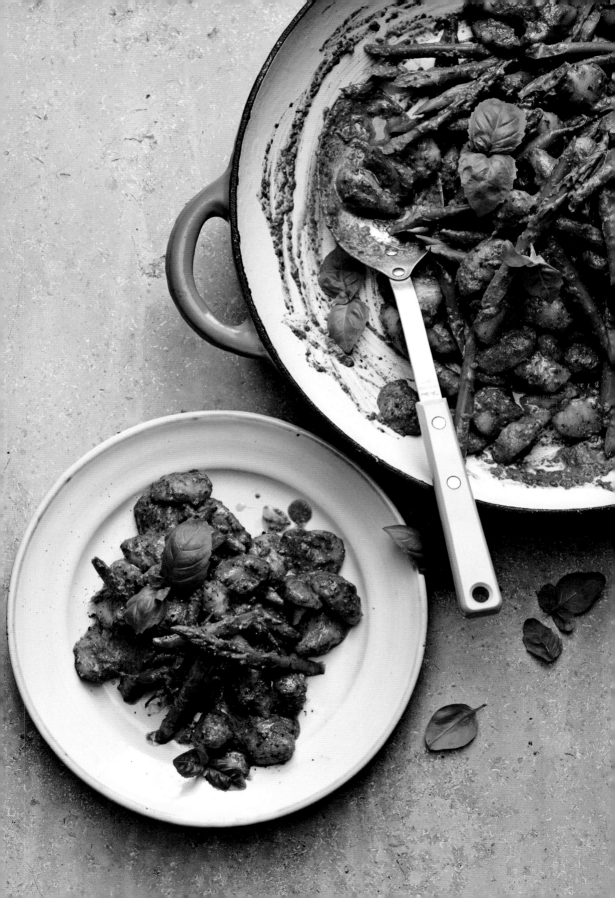

MEDITERRANEAN ORZO

Orzo is essentially a pasta trying to be a grain. But you won't hear us complaining. Here we give it a Mediterranean spin with some of our favourite roasted veggies.

SERVES 4   **DISH** LARGE ROASTING TRAY   **PREP** 15 MINS   **COOK** 25 MINS

500g orzo

1 litre vegetable
  stock

2 courgettes (400g)

2 yellow peppers

1 red onion

1 tbsp dried
  mixed herbs

½ a lemon

salt and pepper

3 garlic cloves

500g cherry
  tomatoes on
  the vine

50g pitted black
  olives

120g jarred
  quartered
  artichokes in
  oil, drained

extra virgin olive oil

a bunch of fresh
  basil (30g)

Preheat the oven to 180°C fan/200°C/gas 6. Put the orzo and vegetable stock into a large roasting tray and stir to combine. Top and tail the courgettes, then cut them into 1cm thick slices. Cut the peppers into 3cm bite-size pieces, and peel and slice the red onion. Spread all the veg on the tray on top of the orzo. Sprinkle with the mixed herbs, the zest from the lemon half, and ½ teaspoon each of salt and pepper. Place the tray in the oven and roast for 15 minutes.

Meanwhile, peel and chop the garlic. Remove the tray from the oven, give everything a gentle stir and sprinkle the garlic all over. Place the tomatoes on top, still on their vines, and roast everything for 10 minutes.

Remove the tray from the oven. Halve the olives and scatter them around the tray, along with the quartered artichokes.

Squeeze the juice from the lemon half all over, and drizzle with 2 tablespoons of extra virgin olive oil. To finish, tear the basil leaves and sprinkle them all over.

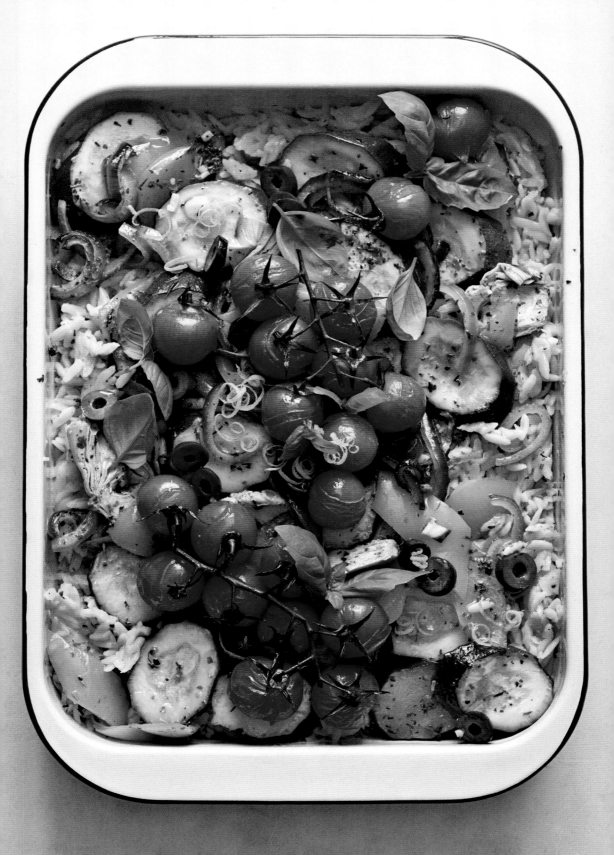

TOFU 'BACON' CAESAR SALAD

Sweet and smoky tofu takes centre stage as the vegan 'bacon' in this salad, which is thrown together with crunchy kale and our creamy cashew-based Caesar dressing.

SERVES 4   **DISH** LARGE ROASTING TRAY   **PREP** 25 MINS   **COOK** 30–35 MINS

400g firm tofu

3 tbsp dark soy sauce

1 tbsp maple syrup

2 tbsp tomato purée

2 tsp smoked paprika

salt and pepper

1 x 400g tin of chickpeas

olive oil

2 little gem lettuces

2 handfuls of chopped kale

1 avocado

For the dressing:

100g cashews

2 tbsp lemon juice

1 garlic clove

1 tsp English mustard

2 tbsp nutritional yeast

2 tsp capers

180ml unsweetened plant-based milk

Preheat the oven to 190°C fan/210°C/gas 6. Line a large roasting tray with baking paper. Drain and press the tofu, if necessary.

To make the marinade, combine the soy sauce, maple syrup, tomato purée, smoked paprika and a large pinch of salt and pepper in a mixing bowl. Crumble the pressed tofu into 1cm pieces straight into the marinade with your hands, toss well, then transfer to one half of the tray.

Drain the chickpeas and put them on the other half of the tray. Sprinkle with a pinch of salt and pepper and drizzle with 1 tablespoon of olive oil. Toss with your hands, then bake for 30–35 minutes, until the chickpeas are crispy, turning everything a couple of times so it cooks evenly.

Meanwhile, put the cashews into a small bowl, cover with hot water straight from the kettle, and leave for 10 minutes. Drain, then put them into a blender with the rest of the dressing ingredients and blend until smooth. Season with salt and pepper to taste.

Remove the tray from the oven. Cut the lettuce into quarters and remove any tough stems from the kale. Place the lettuce and kale on the tray, then pour over most of the dressing and stir everything together.

Pour the remaining dressing into a small bowl to serve. Slice the avocado in half and remove the stone. Then peel the skin, slice the flesh and decorate the salad with the slices.

> Not a fan of tofu? Try substituting a thinly sliced aubergine and roasting it until crispy in the same marinade.

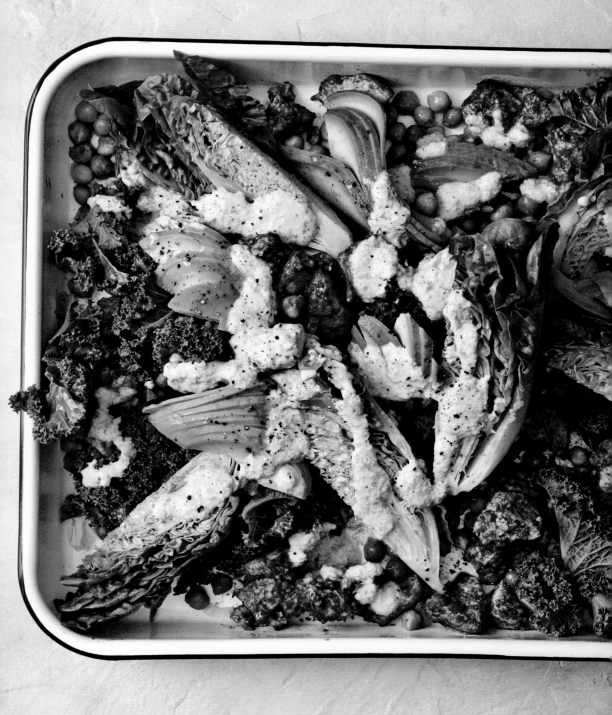

LEMONY LINGUINE

The starch from the linguine adds an extra creaminess to this light, zesty and outrageously easy pasta dish.

SERVES 4   **DISH** LARGE SAUCEPAN   **PREP** 10 MINS   **COOK** 20–22 MINS

olive oil

1 onion

6 garlic cloves

350g cherry tomatoes

1 lemon

100g pitted Kalamata olives

5 tbsp nutritional yeast, plus extra for sprinkling

salt and pepper

400g linguine or spaghetti

200g chopped kale

a small handful of fresh basil

extra virgin olive oil

Heat 2 tablespoons of olive oil in a large saucepan on a medium heat. While the oil heats up, peel and thinly slice the onion, then add to the saucepan and fry for 6 minutes. Peel and thinly slice the garlic, add to the saucepan and fry for 4 minutes until caramelized.

Meanwhile, slice the cherry tomatoes in half, grate the zest from the lemon and slice the olives in half. Add them all to the saucepan along with the nutritional yeast, ½ teaspoon of salt, a large pinch of pepper and 1 litre of hot water straight from the kettle. Give everything a stir, add the linguine to the pan and bring everything to the boil as quickly as possible, then lower the heat and simmer until the pasta is al dente (around 10–12 minutes). Stir every minute or so to prevent the pasta sticking to the bottom of the saucepan.

Remove any large stalks from the kale (save them for your next smoothie) and roughly chop the basil, saving a few leaves for later. Once the pasta is ready, remove it from the heat and stir in the kale, chopped basil and 1 tablespoon of lemon juice, and season to taste with extra salt and pepper, if necessary.

Serve with a sprinkle of nutritional yeast, freshly ground black pepper, the remaining basil leaves and a drizzle of extra virgin olive oil. Deeeeelicious.

Top with your favourite nuts and seeds for some added nutrition.

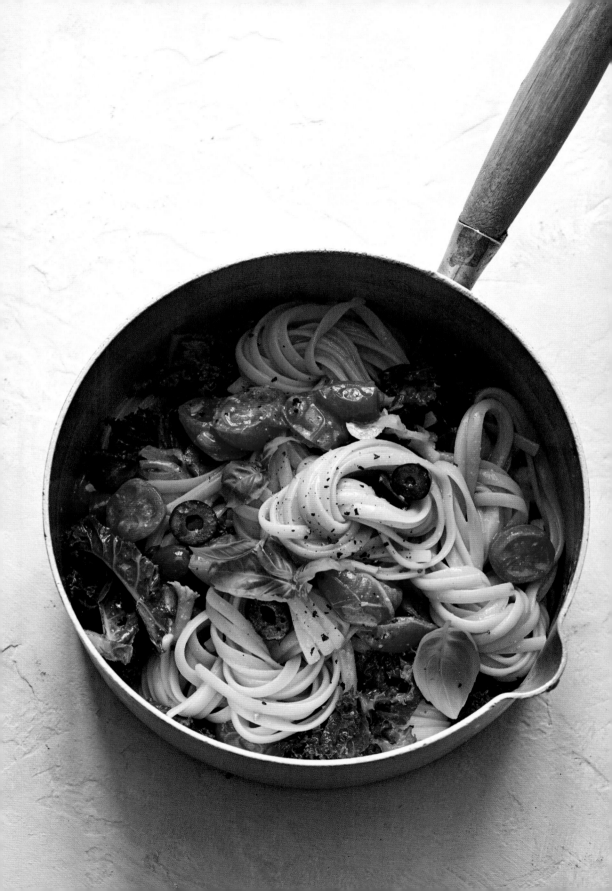

CHEEKY CHIMICHURRI FAJITAS

Our go-to Friday night feast. The fresh chimichurri dressing pairs brilliantly with the roasted veggies, but you can simply sub mashed avocado to make things even easier.

MAKES 8 FAJITAS   **DISH** LARGE ROASTING TRAY   **PREP** 25 MINS   **COOK** 16 MINS

1 red onion

2 tbsp apple cider vinegar

4 portobello mushrooms (250g)

1 red pepper

1 yellow pepper

1 green pepper

1 tbsp smoked paprika

2 tsp ground cumin

¼ tsp cayenne pepper

2 tsp dried oregano

salt and pepper

vegetable oil

8 tortillas

3 tomatoes (270g)

1 lime

For the chimichurri dressing:

6 garlic cloves

1 ripe avocado

1 green chilli

1 lime

extra virgin olive oil

a handful of fresh coriander (15g)

a handful of fresh flat-leaf parsley (15g)

Preheat the oven to 200°C fan/220°C/gas 7. Peel and thinly slice the red onion. Put it into a bowl with the vinegar, stir and set to one side to pickle.

Slice the mushrooms into 1cm-thick strips and slice the peppers into ½cm strips, discarding the seeds and stems. Place them all in a large roasting tray, along with the garlic cloves (skins on), and scatter over the smoked paprika, cumin, cayenne pepper, dried oregano, ½ teaspoon of salt and a large pinch of pepper. Drizzle over 2 tablespoons of vegetable oil, then toss with your hands. Roast in the oven for 16 minutes, stirring halfway.

For the chimichurri, slice the avocado in half, remove the stone, scoop out the flesh and add it to a bowl, then mash with a fork. Finely slice the green chilli, discarding the seeds, and add it to the bowl along with a large pinch of salt, the juice and zest of the lime and 1 tablespoon of extra virgin olive oil. Remove the coriander and parsley leaves from their stalks, finely chop the leaves and stir them into the bowl with 4–6 tablespoons of water. Stir until smooth, adding more water if necessary, then leave to one side.

A minute before the veggies are ready, put the tortillas directly on to a separate oven shelf for 1 minute to warm them through. When everything has finished cooking, remove the garlic cloves from the tray. Peel and finely dice the flesh and add it to the bowl containing the chimichurri. Stir until evenly distributed.

Dice the tomatoes and scatter over the veggies. Slice the lime into quarters and serve with the veggies, alongside the warm tortillas, pickled red onion and chimichurri sauce.

> Add 2 tablespoons of fajita seasoning mix and skip the spices and dried oregano to make things even easier.

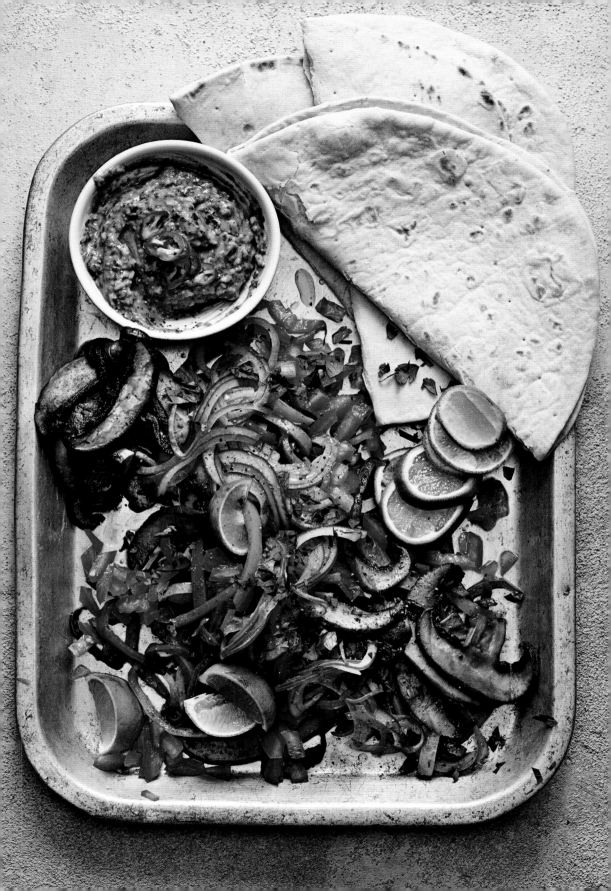

CHEAT'S PIZZA

Spicy, sweet and salty, these perfectly balanced toppings are happy as they are, but don't hesitate to use any leftover veggies to create your own twists.

SERVES 2–4   **DISH** LARGE BAKING TRAY   **PREP** 10 MINS   **COOK** 30–35 MINS

380g pre-rolled vegan puff pastry

6 tbsp passata

¼ tsp dried oregano

salt and pepper

100g cherry tomatoes

100g vegan mozzarella

50g pitted Kalamata olives

1 red chilli

2 tbsp caramelized onion chutney

a small handful of fresh basil (10g)

extra virgin olive oil (optional)

Preheat the oven to 180°C fan/200°C/gas 6. Roll out the pastry on a large baking tray (keep it on top of the baking paper it comes wrapped in) and use a knife to lightly score a 1cm border around the edge, making sure you don't cut all the way through. Then use a fork to prick the inner rectangle half a dozen times to stop it rising in the oven.

Spread the passata evenly over the pastry within the border, then sprinkle over the oregano and season with a large pinch of salt and pepper. Slice the cherry tomatoes in half and scatter them over the passata. Depending on the vegan mozzarella you use, either tear or grate it evenly over the top. Bake in the oven for 20 minutes.

Meanwhile, slice the olives in half and thinly slice the chilli (remove the seeds if you want to dial down the heat). Remove the pizza from the oven, scatter over the olives and sliced chilli, and spoon the chutney evenly over the top. Return the pizza to the oven for 10–15 minutes, or until the pastry is brown and the base is cooked.

Top the pizza with fresh basil leaves, freshly ground black pepper and a drizzle of extra virgin olive oil. How easy was that!

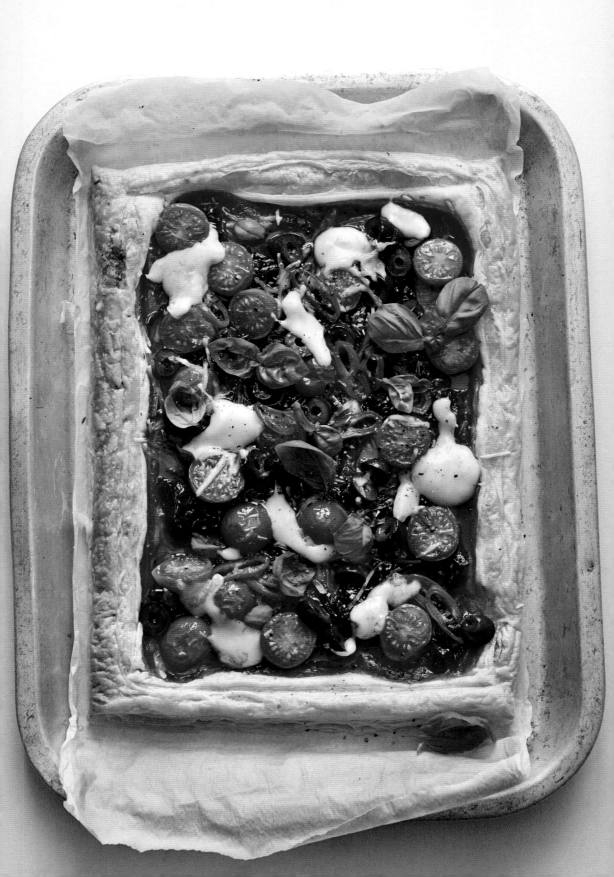

CHICKPEA KOFTE KEBABS

Toasted spices and fresh mint make these vegan koftes light and aromatic. You can also have a go at making your own bread, using the recipe in our Mini Garden Flatbreads (page 42).

SERVES 4   **DISH** FRYING PAN   **PREP** 20 MINS + 1 HR CHILLING   **COOK** 15 MINS

½ tbsp cumin seeds

½ tsp caraway seeds

1 x 400g tin of chickpeas

3 garlic cloves

200g broccoli

½ tsp ground cinnamon

3 tbsp rolled oats

20 fresh mint leaves, plus extra for serving

6 tbsp tahini

4 tsp maple syrup

salt and pepper

olive oil

1 tbsp lemon juice

8 small flatbreads or pittas

250g jarred roasted red peppers, drained

100g mixed salad leaves (spinach, rocket, lettuce)

Place a frying pan over a medium heat. Once hot, toast the cumin and caraway seeds for 3 minutes then transfer to a pestle and mortar, grind to a powder and leave to one side.

Drain and rinse the chickpeas, peel the garlic cloves and break the broccoli into florets. Put them all into a food processor, including any stalks from the broccoli, followed by the toasted spices, ground cinnamon, oats, mint leaves, 2 tablespoons of tahini, 2 teaspoons of maple syrup, ½ teaspoon of salt and a large pinch of pepper. Pulse the ingredients until mostly broken down, but avoid over-processing the ingredients into a mush! The mixture should stick together well in your hands. If not, add a small splash of water.

Divide the mixture into 8. Roll each piece into a thick sausage-like shape about 8cm in length, squeezing the mixture together tightly with your palms as you roll and transferring each kofte to a plate. Refrigerate for at least 1 hour.

When you're ready to cook the kofte, heat 3 tablespoons of olive oil in a frying pan over a medium heat. As soon as the oil is hot, add the kofte and fry for 10–12 minutes carefully turning them every minute or so until golden brown and crispy all over.

For the tahini dressing, combine 4 tablespoons of tahini, 2 teaspoons of maple syrup, 4 tablespoons of cold water and a pinch of salt and pepper in a small bowl. Warm the flatbreads in a toaster and tear the roasted red peppers into strips.

To build the kebabs, place a few strips of roasted red pepper on a warm flatbread, followed by a small handful of salad leaves. Top with the kofte, then drizzle over the tahini dressing and add a couple of mint leaves.

> These kebabs can easily be shaped into burger patties instead! Fry until crispy on both sides and assemble in a burger bun.

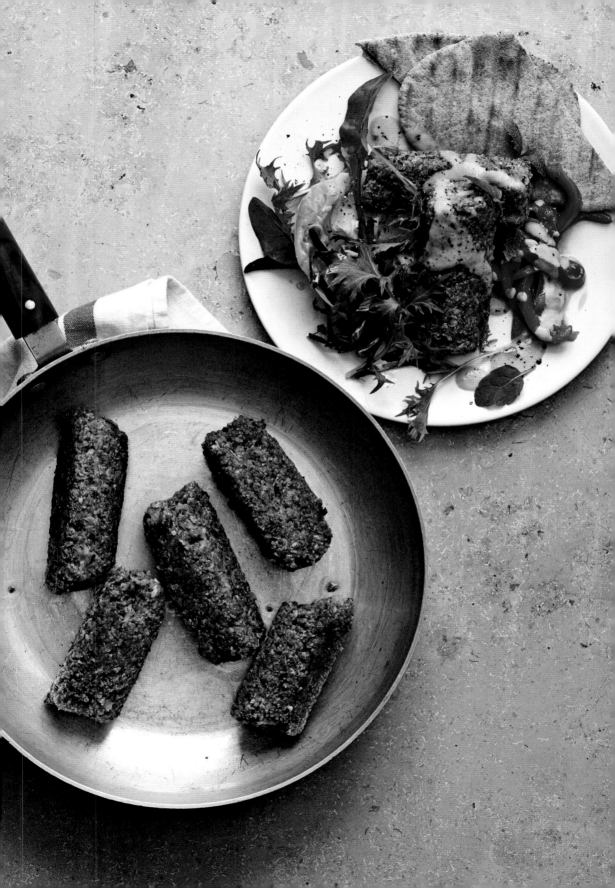

TOFU SATAY WITH CAULIFLOWER RICE

Tofu is packed with protein, so it has become an essential ingredient in our kitchen. Here we serve it with a rich peanut sauce, fresh veggies and cauliflower rice for extra nutrition.

SERVES 4   **DISH** LARGE ROASTING TRAY   **PREP** 20 MINS   **COOK** 25 MINS

550g firm tofu

1 large cauliflower (800g)

vegetable oil

salt and pepper

½ a large cucumber (200g)

150g red cabbage

1 red chilli

1 garlic clove

a thumb of fresh ginger (30g)

1 lime

1 tbsp maple syrup, plus 2 tsp

1 tbsp light soy sauce

4 tbsp smooth peanut butter

1½ tsp chilli garlic sauce

4 tbsp coconut milk, from a tin

2 spring onions

a handful of salted peanuts

Preheat the oven to 200°C fan/220°C/gas 7. Line a large roasting tray with baking paper. Drain and press the tofu, if necessary.

Remove and discard the cauliflower leaves, then break the cauliflower into florets and put them into a food processor (see tip below if you don't have a food processor). Process until the florets have broken down and resemble rice. Put the cauliflower rice on the tray so it takes up two-thirds of the tray.

Cut the tofu into 24 cubes and pierce 6 pieces on to a skewer. Repeat until you have 4 skewers, then transfer them to the remaining space in the tray. Drizzle the cauliflower and tofu with 2 tablespoons of vegetable oil, and season well with salt and pepper. Give both a gentle toss, then bake in the oven for 25 minutes, stirring the cauliflower and turning the tofu halfway through.

Meanwhile, slice the cucumber and thinly slice the cabbage and half the red chilli (saving the other half for later). Peel and chop the garlic and ginger. Put everything into a mixing bowl along with the juice from half of the lime, 2 teaspoons of maple syrup and a pinch of salt. Stir to combine, then set to one side so the veggies pickle.

Next, prepare the satay sauce by combining the soy sauce with the peanut butter, the juice of the remaining lime half, 1 tablespoon of maple syrup, the chilli garlic sauce and the coconut milk.

Remove the tray from the oven and brush the satay sauce all over the tofu skewers. Add the pickled veggies to the tray. Slice the spring onions and the remaining red chilli, roughly chop the salted peanuts, then sprinkle them all over the tray. Pour any remaining satay sauce into a small bowl to serve.

> Don't have a food processor? Simply use a hand-held grater to coarsely grate the cauliflower into 'rice'.

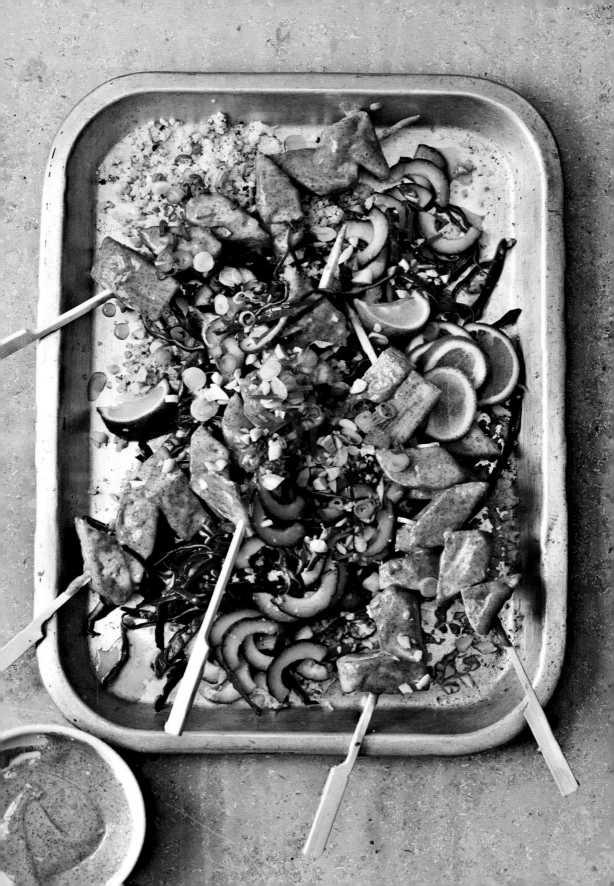

SWEET POTATO THAI GREEN CURRY

Thailand has a special place in our hearts. The people, the history and, of course . . . the food, always so fresh and full of flavour, which we capture in this gorgeous curry.

SERVES 4   **DISH** WOK   **PREP** 30 MINS   **COOK** 35 MINS

2 large sweet
potatoes (600g)

1 large potato (400g)

1 tbsp coconut oil

2 shallots

4 garlic cloves

a thumb of fresh
ginger (30g)

2 green bird's-eye
chillies

a bunch of fresh
coriander (30g)

5 kaffir lime leaves

2 lemongrass stalks

1 tsp ground cumin

1 x 400g tin of
coconut milk

500ml vegetable
stock

2 tbsp soy sauce

1 red pepper

100g mangetout

½ a lime

a handful of Thai
basil

Peel and dice all the potatoes and cut into 2–3cm chunks. Put the coconut oil into a wok over a medium-high heat. Once the oil is hot, add the potatoes and fry for 10–15 minutes, or until they begin to brown.

Meanwhile, prepare the curry paste: peel and roughly chop the shallots, garlic and ginger, then put them into a food processor (see tip below if you don't have a food processor). Roughly chop the chillies, coriander and kaffir lime leaves. Remove and discard the tough outer layers of the lemongrass, then add everything to the food processor along with the cumin. Process until mostly broken down.

Reduce the heat under the wok to medium. Add 4 tablespoons of coconut milk along with the curry paste, and fry for 5 minutes.

Stir in the rest of the coconut milk, the stock and soy sauce, and bring to the boil. Then reduce the heat and simmer for 5 minutes.

Meanwhile, slice the pepper into ½cm strips, discarding the seeds and stems, then add to the wok along with the mangetout. Simmer for 5–8 minutes, or until the potatoes are soft and the other veggies are still slightly crunchy. Remove the pan from the heat and stir in the juice of the lime. Finally, decorate with a few Thai basil leaves.

> Don't have a food processor? Finely chop the shallots, garlic, ginger, chillies, kaffir lime leaves and lemongrass, and add them to a pestle and mortar. Grind them until mostly broken down, then add the cumin and coriander, and grind into a paste.

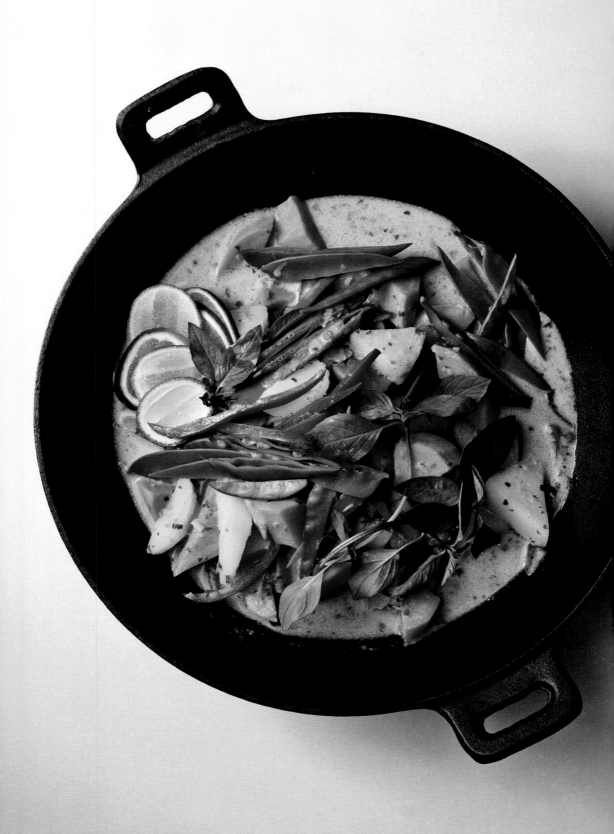

ROASTED SQUASH, CAULIFLOWER + SAGE

Fresh sage is a seriously underrated herb, and there's no better pairing for it than butternut squash, which makes this Europe-meets-Middle East fusion dish a total experience.

SERVES 4   **DISH** LARGE ROASTING TRAY   **PREP** 25 MINS   **COOK** 40 MINS

1 butternut squash (approx 1.2kg)

1 large cauliflower (750g)

2 red onions

salt and pepper

1 tsp nutmeg

olive oil

1 x 400g tin of green lentils

12 fresh sage leaves

160g baby spinach

1 lemon

4 tbsp tahini

1 tbsp Dijon mustard

½ tbsp maple syrup

40g pecans

1 pomegranate

Preheat the oven to 180°C fan/200°C/gas 6. Cut the butternut squash in half lengthways, peel the skin, spoon out the seeds, then slice the flesh into 1cm thick semicircles. Remove the leaves from the cauliflower and slice the cauliflower through the stem into 2cm thick 'steaks'. Cut the red onions into quarters, leaving the skins on.

Put the squash, cauliflower and red onions into a large roasting tray, season generously with salt and pepper, sprinkle with nutmeg, then drizzle with 3 tablespoons of olive oil. Rub the seasoning evenly over the veggies, then roast for 30 minutes.

Remove the tray from the oven. Drain and rinse the lentils and add them to the tray. Roughly chop the sage leaves and sprinkle them over the veggies, then spread the spinach across the tray. Put back into the oven and roast for 10 minutes.

Meanwhile, zest the lemon and leave to one side. Prepare the tahini dressing by combining the tahini with the Dijon mustard, maple syrup, 1 tablespoon of lemon juice and 4 tablespoons of water in a small mixing bowl until smooth and runny. Taste and season to your liking. Note: you may need more water or more tahini to get the perfect consistency, depending on which brand of tahini you use.

Roughly chop the pecans. Cut the pomegranate in half and whack the skin of each half with a wooden spoon to ease the seeds out. Remove the tray from the oven and squeeze the rest of the lemon juice on top. Drizzle the tahini dressing around the tray, sprinkle over the pecans and pomegranate seeds, and finish with a scattering of lemon zest.

> Not a fan of pomegranate? Sub with a handful of pitted and halved grapes.

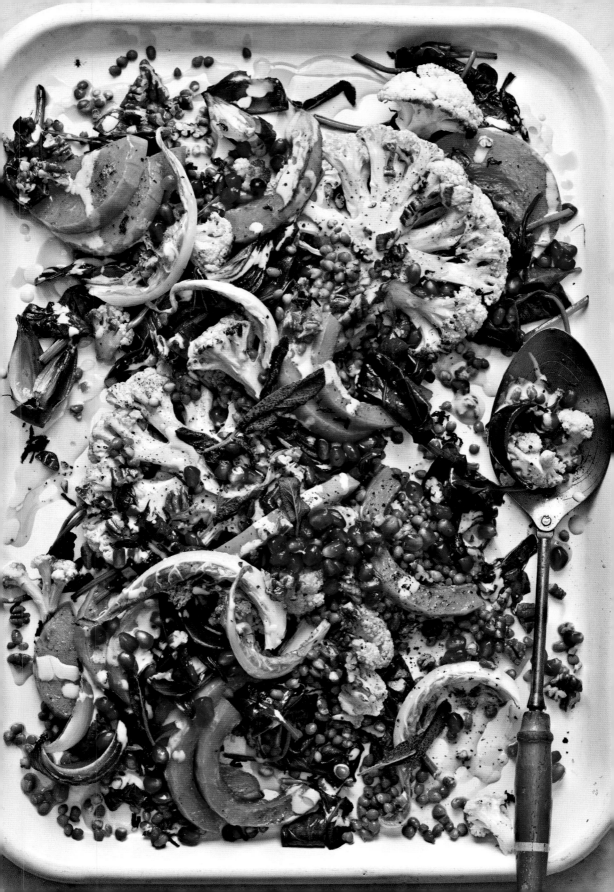

AUBERGINE + COURGETTE BAKE

Wholesome and hearty. The fennel seeds give this vegetable bake a lovely warm fragrance, which marries well with the rich tomato sauce. Goes well with a simple side salad.

SERVES 4 **DISH** SHALLOW OVENPROOF CASSEROLE PAN **PREP** 25 MINS **COOK** 1 HR

olive oil

1 leek

1 aubergine

3 courgettes (600g)

5 garlic cloves

8 sprigs of fresh thyme

70g pitted Kalamata olives

½ tsp fennel seeds, plus an extra pinch

¼ tsp chilli flakes

2 x 400g tin of chopped tomatoes

1 tbsp balsamic vinegar

salt and pepper

40g dried breadcrumbs

Heat 2 tablespoons of olive oil in a shallow ovenproof casserole pan on a medium heat. While the oil heats up, slice the leek into ½cm-thick pieces, then add to the pan and fry for 10–15 minutes until soft.

Meanwhile, top and tail the aubergine and 2 of the courgettes, and dice both. Peel and chop 4 garlic cloves, and add to the pan along with the aubergine and courgette. Fry for 5 minutes.

Pick the leaves off 6 sprigs of thyme, halve the Kalamata olives, and add both to the pan along with the fennel seeds, chilli flakes, tomatoes, balsamic vinegar, and generous pinches of salt and pepper. Give everything a good stir, bring to the boil, then reduce the heat and simmer for 8 minutes.

Preheat the oven to 180°C fan/200°C/gas 6. Slice the remaining courgette lengthways into ½cm-thick slices and use to decorate the top of the bake. Sprinkle the slices with salt and pepper, and drizzle with olive oil.

Put the breadcrumbs into a small mixing bowl along with pinches of salt and pepper and 2 teaspoons of olive oil. Pick the leaves off the remaining 2 thyme sprigs, peel and chop the remaining garlic clove, and add both to the bowl, along with an extra pinch of fennel seeds. Stir to combine, then sprinkle the breadcrumb mixture all over the top of the bake. Cook for 30–35 minutes, or until the breadcrumbs are golden brown. Delicious.

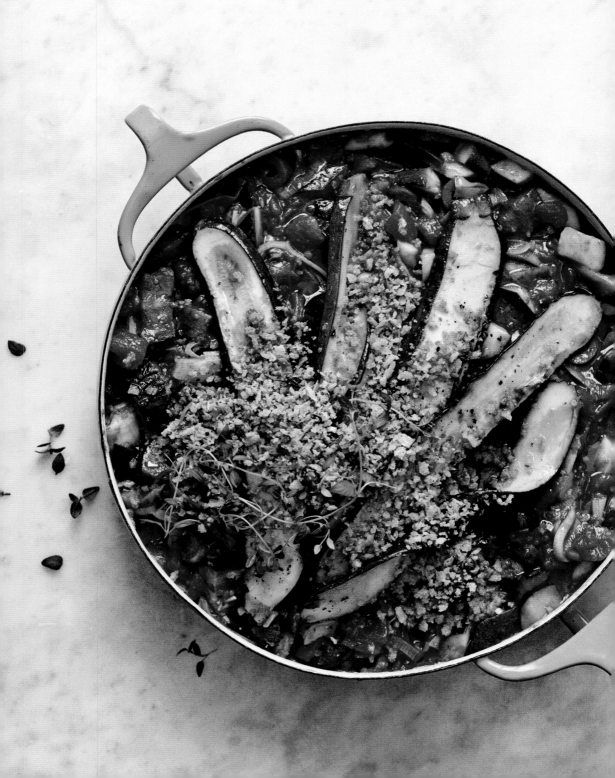

CARIBBEAN FEAST

Feast your eyes on this. It's a sweet, spicy and savoury fiesta of food, where our very own DIY jerk sauce teams up with fresh fruits and veggies to create a carnival of flavours.

SERVES 4 **DISH** LARGE ROASTING TRAY **PREP** 25 MINS **COOK** 40 MINS

200g basmati rice

1 x 400g tin of
coconut milk

1 x 400g tin of kidney
beans

salt and pepper

4 corn on the cob

300g oyster
mushrooms

2 ripe plantains

⅛ of a Savoy cabbage

⅛ of a red cabbage

1 lime

3 tbsp vegan
mayonnaise

1 ripe mango

a handful of fresh
coriander (15g)

For the jerk marinade:

2 shallots

a thumb of fresh
ginger (30g)

6 garlic cloves

1 Scotch bonnet chilli

8 sprigs of fresh
thyme

2 tbsp light soy sauce

1 tbsp maple syrup

1 tbsp ground allspice

1 tsp ground
cinnamon

vegetable oil

First prepare the jerk marinade. Peel and roughly chop the shallots, ginger and garlic, and put them into a food processor (see tip below if you don't have a food processor). Remove the stalk from the Scotch bonnet, cut in half and discard the seeds, then pick the leaves off the thyme and add both to the food processor along with the soy sauce, maple syrup, juice from half the lime, allspice, cinnamon, 3 tablespoons of vegetable oil and pinches of salt and pepper.

Preheat the oven to 200°C fan/220°C/gas 7. Put the rice into a sieve and rinse until the water runs clear, then transfer to a large roasting tray along with the coconut milk, 250ml of water and pinches of salt and pepper. Drain and rinse the kidney beans and add them to the tray, then stir to combine. Cut the sweetcorn cobs in half, rub 4 tablespoons of the jerk marinade all over them, and add them to the tray. Cover the tray with baking paper or a larger tray, and roast for 15 minutes.

Meanwhile, tear any large mushrooms in half and rub them with the remaining marinade. Peel the plantains, cut them into 1cm-thick slices, put them into a bowl, season with salt and pepper and drizzle with olive oil. Remove the baking paper from the tray and discard, then add the mushrooms and plantains to the tray, covering the rice to help it steam. Bake uncovered for 20–25 minutes, turning the plantain and mushrooms halfway.

Meanwhile, prepare the slaw by finely chopping the Savoy and red cabbage. Put both into a mixing bowl along with the juice from the remaining lime half and the vegan mayonnaise. Stir to combine and set to one side.

To serve, top the Caribbean feast with the slaw, then peel and dice the mango and scatter over the tray along with the coriander leaves.

> Don't have a food processor? Finely chop the shallots, ginger, garlic and Scotch bonnet and add them to a pestle and mortar. Grind until mostly broken down. Add the thyme leaves along with the remaining ingredients and 3 tablespoons of vegetable oil. Grind into a rough paste.

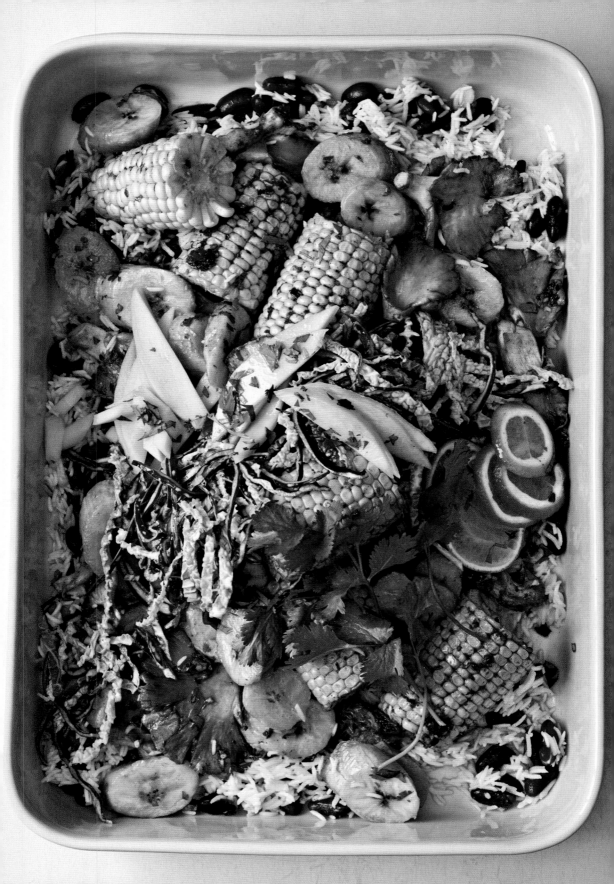

SWEET + SOUR JACKFRUIT FAKEAWAY

Jackfruit has a lovely subtle sweetness and it's a brilliant meat replacer in vegan cooking. We pair it with sweet and sour flavours to create our one-tray twist on this classic Chinese takeaway.

SERVES 4   **DISH** LARGE ROASTING TRAY   **PREP** 25 MINS   **COOK** 50–60 MINS

2 x 560g tins of
  jackfruit in brine

salt and pepper

vegetable oil

300g basmati rice

3 peppers (we use
  red, yellow and
  orange)

1 onion

1 x 425g tin of
  pineapple chunks
  in juice

2 spring onions

a handful of sesame
  seeds

For the sauce:

6 tbsp tomato
  ketchup

3 tbsp cornflour

2 tbsp light soy sauce

3 tbsp maple syrup

2 tbsp apple cider
  vinegar

¼ tsp chilli powder

400ml pineapple
  juice

Preheat the oven to 200°C fan/220°C/gas 7. Drain and rinse the jackfruit, pat dry with kitchen paper or a tea towel, then put it on a large roasting tray, season with salt and pepper and generously drizzle with 1½ tablespoons of vegetable oil. Toss with your hands, then roast for 20–25 minutes or until slightly charred around the edges. Remove the jackfruit from the tray and leave in a bowl to one side.

Drain and rinse the rice, then put it on the tray along with 450ml of water and a pinch of salt. Stir to combine, then cover with baking paper or another large tray and roast for 15 minutes.

Meanwhile, whisk together the sauce ingredients in a mixing bowl. Next, prep the veggies: cut the peppers into 3cm cubes, discarding the seeds and stalks, then peel the onion and cut into 8 wedges.

Remove the tray from the oven and discard the baking paper. Using a spoon, move the rice over so it takes up a quarter of the tray and pour 150ml of cold water over it. Drain the tinned pineapple and add it to the remaining three-quarters of the tray along with the jackfruit, veggies and sauce. Give the sauce and veggies a gentle stir, then roast for 15–20 minutes.

To finish, roughly chop the spring onions and sprinkle on top, along with the sesame seeds.

> Lots of supermarkets now stock tinned jackfruit, but if you're having trouble finding it simply sub with sliced tofu and follow the same method.

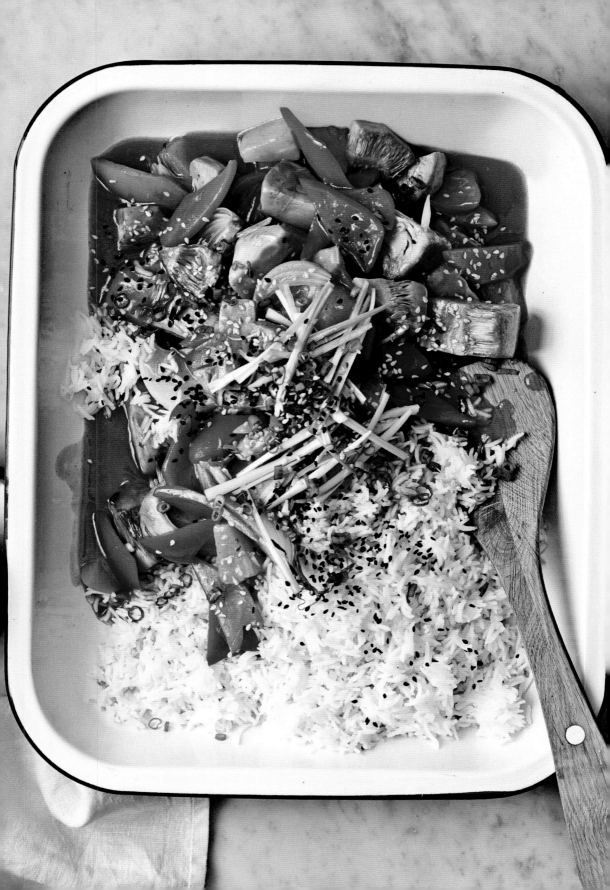

'FISHCAKES' WITH HOMEMADE SLAW + MAYO

Nori is our secret weapon in this dish. It helps to recreate that salty taste of the sea, and you'll now find it in most big supermarkets.

MAKES 4 FISHCAKES   **DISH** FRYING PAN   **PREP** 25 MINS   **COOK** 10–15 MINS

1 tbsp ground chia seeds

2 x 400g tins of chickpeas

6 spring onions

3 garlic cloves

4 sheets of nori

a large handful of fresh flat-leaf parsley (20g), plus extra for serving

a large handful of fresh dill (20g), plus extra for serving

2 lemons

salt and pepper

75ml unsweetened plant-based milk

75g dried breadcrumbs

vegetable oil

To serve:

200g silken tofu

1 tsp English mustard

200g celeriac

1 Pink Lady apple

a handful of mixed salad leaves (rocket, spinach, radicchio)

Put the chia seeds into a small bowl, stir in 2 tablespoons of water and set to one side to create a chia 'egg'.

Drain and rinse the chickpeas, then put them into a food processor. Trim the spring onions and roughly chop them, peel the garlic cloves, tear the nori into smaller pieces, and add everything to the food processor along with the parsley and dill, the zest and juice of half a lemon, ½ teaspoon each of salt and pepper and finally the chia egg from earlier. Process until the mixture comes together but still has some texture, then shape into 4 fishcakes.

Put the milk into a small bowl and the breadcrumbs into a separate bowl. Dip the fishcakes first into the milk, then into the breadcrumbs. Heat 3–4 tablespoons of vegetable oil in a frying pan on a medium heat and fry the fishcakes for 5 minutes on each side, or until golden.

Meanwhile, for the mayonnaise, rinse out the food processor, then put in the silken tofu, 1 tablespoon of lemon juice, the English mustard, pinches of salt and pepper and 4 tablespoons of vegetable oil and blend until smooth. For the slaw, peel the celeriac and thinly slice it along with the apple. Put both into a serving bowl, season with salt and pepper, stir in 4 tablespoons of the mayo and top with a few parsley leaves.

To serve, cut the remaining lemon into wedges and serve alongside the fishcakes, slaw and salad leaves with an extra sprinkling of dill. Transfer the remaining mayo to a small bowl, to serve with the fishcakes.

> If you're in a rush, skip the homemade mayo and use one of the shop-bought vegan versions, which are now readily available in supermarkets.

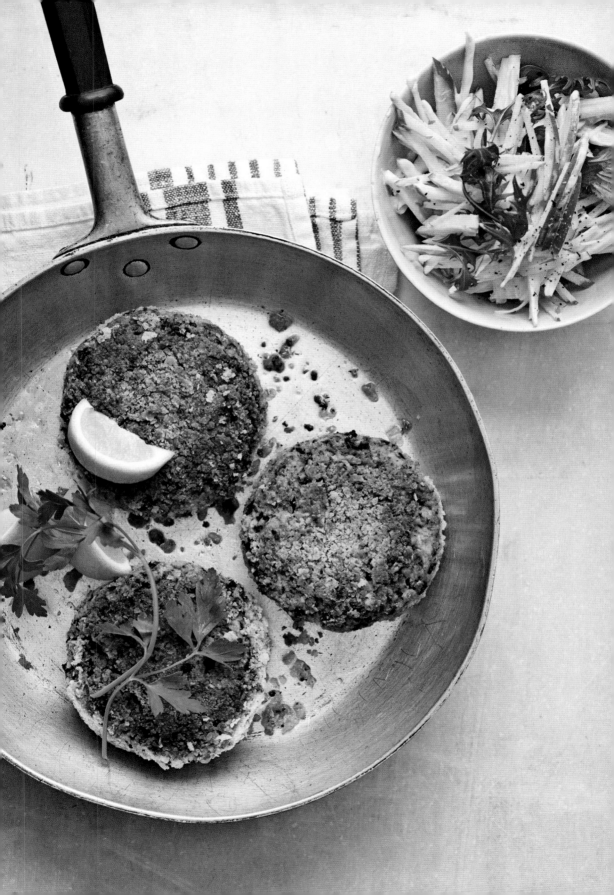

COURGETTE CANNELLONI WITH TOFU RICOTTA

Whodathunkit? Before we were vegan we never dreamed that one day we'd be creating 'ricotta' using tofu. We usually serve this cannelloni with a simple side salad.

SERVES 4   **DISH** OVENDISH   **PREP** 25 MINS   **COOK** 30 MINS

400g firm tofu

2 sprigs of fresh
   rosemary

800g passata

salt and pepper

1 lemon

3 tablespoons
   nutritional yeast

50g spinach

½ tsp nutmeg

olive oil

2 garlic cloves

2–3 medium
   courgettes (about
   500g)

4 tbsp vegan pesto

crusty bread,
   to serve

Preheat the oven to 180°C fan/200°C/gas 6. Drain and press the tofu, if necessary. Pick the leaves off the rosemary sprigs and finely chop them, then put them into an oven dish. Pour the passata into the dish, along with a pinch of salt and pepper, and give everything a good stir.

Next start preparing the tofu ricotta. Break the tofu up in a food processor (see tip below if you don't have a food processor), along with the juice from the lemon, the nutritional yeast, ½ teaspoon of salt, a large pinch of pepper, the spinach, nutmeg and 2 tablespoons of olive oil. Peel the garlic and add the cloves to the food processor, then process until smooth.

Using a mandolin or a knife, slice the courgettes into 2mm-thick strips until you have 24 strips. Scoop a generously heaped teaspoon's worth of the tofu ricotta on to a courgette strip, roll into a cannelloni-style tube, then transfer it to the dish seam-side down. Repeat until you've created 24 tubes, placing them close together in the dish. Lightly brush the tops of the tubes with olive oil, then cook in the oven for 30 minutes.

To serve, drizzle the vegan pesto over the top and pair the cannelloni with slices of crusty bread. Heaven.

> Don't have a food processor? Simply break the tofu into small pieces using your hands. Then add the juice from the lemon, nutritional yeast, salt and pepper, nutmeg and olive oil. Peel and dice the garlic, and finely chop the spinach. Add them in and give everything a good stir.

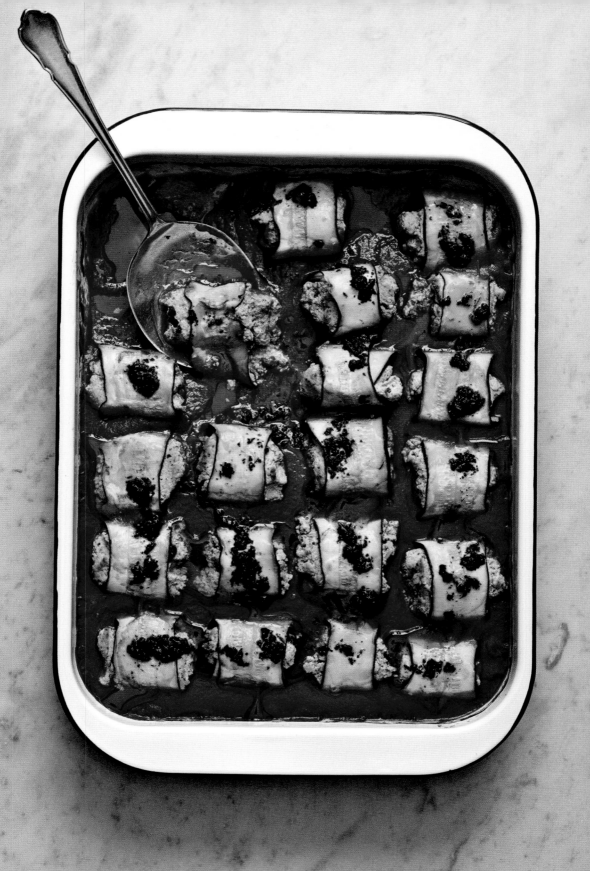

'CHICKEN' SUPREME

It turns out fried oyster mushrooms have an uncanny resemblance to chicken, so we combine them with a rich, robust and creamy roux to create this supremely tasty dinner.

SERVES 4   **DISH** SHALLOW CASSEROLE PAN   **PREP** 20 MINS   **COOK** 40 MINS

500g oyster
   mushrooms

3 tbsp vegan
   margarine

1½ tbsp chicken
   seasoning mix

6 shallots

3 garlic cloves

3 tbsp plain flour

200ml dry white wine

500ml vegetable
   stock

1 tsp Dijon mustard

1 tsp herbes de
   Provence

200g green beans

a small handful
   of fresh
   chives (10g)

a large handful
   of fresh flat-leaf
   parsley (20g)

250ml vegan
   single cream

salt and pepper

sliced baguette,
   to serve

Slice the oyster mushrooms into 1cm strips. Melt 2 tablespoons of the vegan margarine in a shallow casserole pan over a medium-high heat, then add the mushrooms, stir in the chicken seasoning and fry for 15–20 minutes, or until the mushrooms are crispy. Remove from the heat, spoon the mushrooms on to a plate and keep to one side.

Meanwhile, peel and chop the shallots and garlic. Melt the remaining tablespoon of vegan margarine in the pan, reduce the heat to medium, then add the shallots and garlic. Fry for 4 minutes, stirring occasionally. Stir in the flour and fry for 2 minutes, then very slowly pour in the wine, stirring quickly to prevent the flour clumping together and using the wine to deglaze the pan, gathering up as much flavour as possible. Simmer for 1–2 minutes, then stir in the stock, mustard and herbes de Provence. Trim the ends off the green beans and add them to the pan. Simmer for 10 minutes, until the beans are cooked but still have a good bite left to them.

Meanwhile, chop the chives and pick the parsley leaves from their stalks, then roughly chop the leaves. Add the cooked mushrooms, most of the parsley leaves and the vegan single cream to the pan, and cook through for 1–2 minutes. Season to taste with salt and pepper.

Top with the chopped chives, the remaining parsley leaves and freshly ground black pepper, and serve alongside the sliced baguette.

If you want to avoid using the white wine, simply substitute 2 teaspoons of apple cider vinegar.

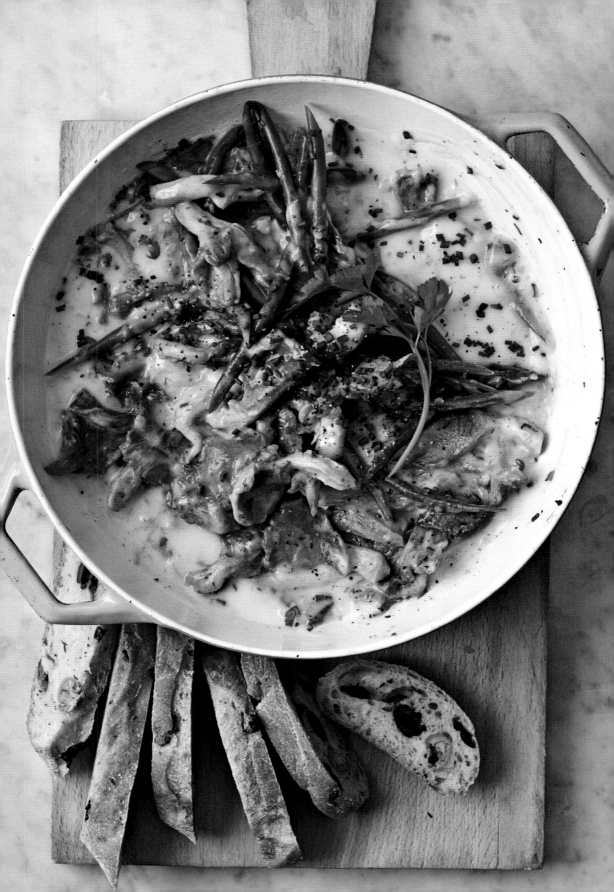

HARISSA-SPICED AUBERGINE

Cooking hearty, nutritious and comforting food can be super easy. Here we throw together pulses and veggies with harissa paste for a substantial meal that doesn't hold back on flavour.

SERVES 4   **DISH** OVENDISH   **PREP** 15 MINS   **COOK** 40 MINS

2 aubergines (580g)

3 tbsp rose harissa

vegetable oil

salt and pepper

2 shallots

3 garlic cloves

1 x 400g tin of chickpeas

2 bell peppers (we use red and yellow)

200g ready-to-eat Puy lentils

1 x 400g tin of chopped tomatoes

200ml vegetable stock

vegan plain yoghurt

a small handful of fresh mint leaves

1 tbsp toasted almond flakes

Preheat the oven to 180°C fan/200°C/gas 6. Cut the aubergines in half lengthways and criss-cross the flesh. In a small bowl, combine the harissa paste with 2 tablespoons of vegetable oil and pinches of salt and pepper, then rub a teaspoon's worth over the cut side of each aubergine half (save the remaining harissa mix for later). Place the aubergines in an oven dish and bake for 20 minutes.

Meanwhile, peel and chop the shallots and garlic, drain and rinse the chickpeas, deseed the peppers and thinly slice them.

Remove the dish from the oven and take out the aubergines. Add the shallots, garlic, chickpeas, lentils, peppers, tinned tomatoes, stock, the harissa mix from earlier, and pinches of salt and pepper to the dish. Give everything a good stir, then put the aubergines back on top and bake for 20 minutes.

To finish, top with a few spoonfuls of vegan yoghurt, a few mint leaves and the toasted almond flakes.

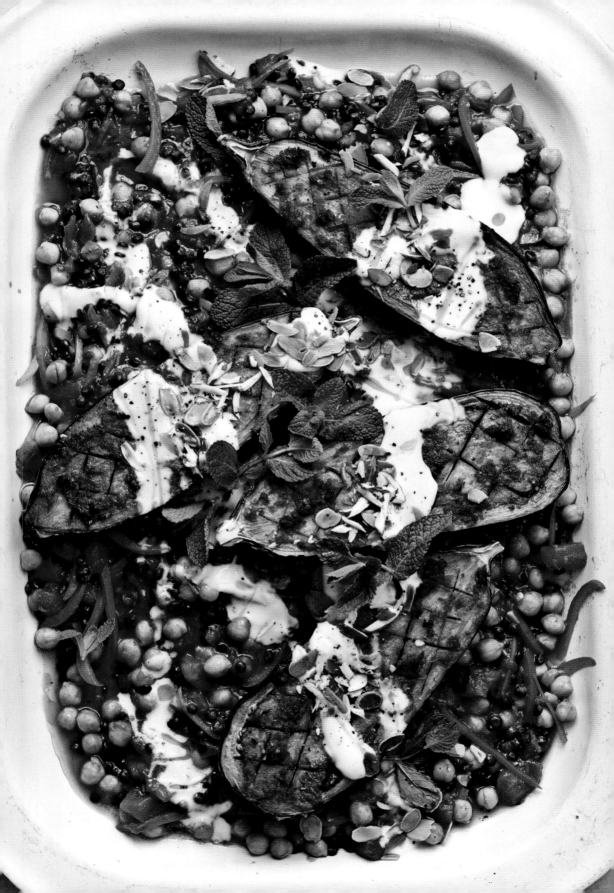

LAZY LASAGNE

Lasagnes are the real deal but we rarely have the time to create them at home. Step forward our 'no fuss' version, aka the perfect midweek meal when only a lasagne will do.

SERVES 4–5 **DISH** SHALLOW OVENPROOF CASSEROLE PAN **PREP** 25 MINS **COOK** 1 HR

1 onion

2 sticks of celery

2 carrots

olive oil

400g closed-cup mushrooms

4 garlic cloves

3 large sprigs of fresh rosemary

300ml red wine

2 x 400g tins of chopped tomatoes

2 tbsp brown rice miso paste

4 tsp dried oregano

salt and pepper

200g lasagne sheets

100g vegan cheese

80g walnuts

Finely chop the onion, celery and carrots. Drizzle 3 tablespoons of olive oil into a shallow ovenproof casserole pan on a medium-high heat and once hot, fry the veggies for 10 minutes. Meanwhile, finely chop the mushrooms and peel and chop the garlic, then add both to the pan and fry for 10 minutes.

Pick the leaves off the sprigs of rosemary and finely chop them, then add them to the pan along with the wine. Simmer for a few minutes to reduce, then add the chopped tomatoes, miso paste, 2 teaspoons of oregano, and generous pinches of salt and pepper. Bring the mixture to the boil, then reduce the heat and simmer for 10 minutes.

Preheat the oven to 180°C fan/200°C/gas 6. Break up the lasagne sheets and add them to the pan at random, tucking them in and under the sauce. Pull out the corners of a few of the sheets so they pop out above the sauce. Now grate the cheese all over the top. Finely chop the walnuts and put them into a small bowl along with the other 2 teaspoons of oregano, 2 teaspoons of olive oil and pinches of salt and pepper. Stir to combine, then sprinkle over the cheese. Bake for 25–30 minutes, or until the top is golden.

> We can confirm that this tastes even better the next day.

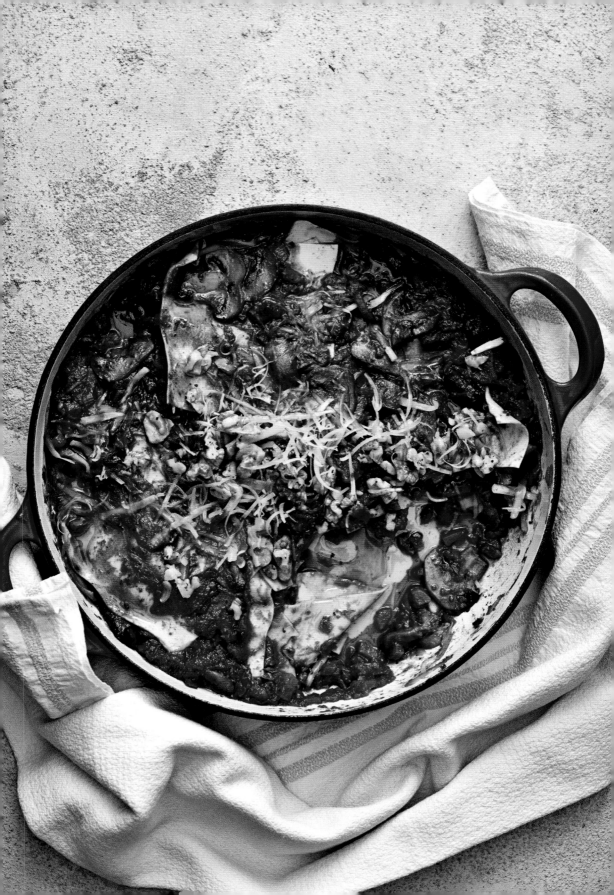

ALMOND + CHICKPEA CURRY

You know those staple recipes you recreate week in and week out and they simply never get boring? This creamy and nutritious curry is one that we return to again and again.

SERVES 3–4   **DISH** CASSEROLE POT   **PREP** 15 MINS   **COOK** 40 MINS

2 onions

1 tbsp coconut oil

4 fresh red chillies

6 garlic cloves

a thumb of fresh ginger (30g)

1½ tbsp medium curry powder

½ tsp fennel seeds

1 tsp ground fenugreek

2 x 400g tins of chickpeas

1 x 400g tin of plum tomatoes

1 x 400g tin of full fat coconut milk

50g ground almonds

salt and pepper

2 handfuls of baby spinach

1 tsp maple syrup

½ a lime

vegan naans, to serve

Peel and slice the onions. Put the coconut oil into a casserole pot on a medium heat. When the oil is hot, add the onion to the pan along with the whole red chillies and fry for 8 minutes.

Peel and chop the garlic and ginger, then add both to the pot along with the curry powder, fennel seeds and fenugreek, and fry for 2 minutes. Drain and rinse the chickpeas, then add them to the pot with the plum tomatoes, coconut milk, ground almonds, and large pinches of salt and pepper. Give everything a good stir and bring the curry to the boil, then reduce the heat and simmer for 30 minutes, stirring occasionally.

Add the spinach, maple syrup and the juice of the half lime, and stir until the spinach has wilted. Taste, then season to your liking with salt and pepper. Toast the naans to serve.

> This curry is perfect for batch cooking. Freeze it in airtight containers and save for an evening when you simply don't have the energy to cook.

MUSHROOM STROGANOFF

Simple ingredients with big results. This stroganoff delivers exactly what it needs to. Creamy, salty, slightly sharp and super fresh, there's something here for everyone.

SERVES 4   **DISH** CASSEROLE POT   **PREP** 10 MINS   **COOK** 30–35 MINS

1 onion

olive oil

4 garlic cloves

a bunch of fresh
    flat-leaf parsley
    (30g)

500g chestnut
    mushrooms

salt and pepper

2 tsp paprika

½ tsp chilli powder

2 tsp Dijon mustard

1 tbsp light soy sauce

1 litre vegetable
    stock

400g tagliatelle

250ml vegan single
    cream

½ a lemon

Peel and chop the onion. Put 2 tablespoons of olive oil into a casserole pot over a medium heat. As soon as it's hot, add the onion and fry for 6 minutes, stirring occasionally. Meanwhile, peel and chop the garlic and pick the parsley leaves off their stalks. Finely chop the parsley stalks and thinly slice the mushrooms.

Add the garlic and parsley stalks to the pot, and fry for 2 minutes. Then turn the heat up to medium-high and add the mushrooms, along with a pinch of salt and pepper. Fry for 10 minutes, stirring occasionally.

Stir in the paprika and chilli powder, and cook for 2 minutes. Then add the mustard, soy sauce and stock. Give everything a stir, add the pasta and bring to the boil, then lower the heat and simmer with the lid on for 10–15 minutes, or until the pasta is al dente. Give the pasta a stir every couple of minutes to prevent it sticking to the bottom of the pot.

Meanwhile, roughly chop the parsley leaves. When the pasta is ready, stir in most of the parsley leaves along with the vegan single cream and the juice of the lemon half. Cook through for a minute, then serve the stroganoff topped with the remaining parsley and a sprinkling of pepper.

AUBERGINE KEBABS WITH TZATZIKI + CHILLI

One of Ben's old guilty pleasures was a late-night doner kebab. Nowadays we make kebabs at home using fresh ingredients, aromatic spices and . . . they're made entirely from plants.

SERVES 4   **DISH** GRIDDLE PAN   **PREP** 20 MINS   **COOK** 45 MINS

vegetable oil

2 aubergines (550g)

4 tbsp tomato purée

2 tsp ras el hanout

2 tsp maple syrup

salt and pepper

For the tzatziki:

½ of a cucumber (150g)

1 garlic clove

a handful of fresh mint leaves

5 tbsp vegan plain yoghurt

1 lemon

For the chilli topping:

200g jarred roasted red peppers

¼ tsp chilli flakes

To serve:

4 medium flatbreads

1 red onion

2 ripe tomatoes

jarred pickled red cabbage

4 jarred green chilli peppers

Preheat the oven to a low temperature, ready to keep the flatbreads warm. Drizzle 1 tablespoon of vegetable oil into a griddle pan on a medium heat. Once the pan is hot, toast the flatbreads one at a time for 1–2 minutes on each side.

Meanwhile, top and tail the aubergines and cut them into 3cm cubes. Put the tomato purée, ras el hanout, maple syrup, pinches of salt and pepper and 2 tablespoons of vegetable oil into a large bowl. Stir to combine, then throw in the pieces of aubergine and toss them with your hands until fully coated.

Remove the flatbreads from the griddle pan as they are ready, and put them into the oven to keep warm, laying them directly on the oven shelf. Add a little more oil to the pan, then add the aubergine pieces and fry for 15 minutes (in batches if necessary), turning them every few minutes.

Meanwhile, prepare the tzatziki. Dice the cucumber, peel and chop the garlic, finely chop a small handful of mint leaves (saving some to decorate with later), and put it all into a small mixing bowl along with the vegan yoghurt, 1 tablespoon of lemon juice and small pinches of salt and pepper. Stir to combine.

For the chilli topping, finely chop the roasted red peppers and put them into a small mixing bowl with the chilli flakes, pinches of salt and pepper and 1 tablespoon of lemon juice. Stir to combine. Peel and slice the red onion. Slice the tomatoes and jarred green chilli peppers.

To serve, divide the aubergine between the flatbreads and top with spoonfuls of tzatziki, slices of red onion and tomato, handfuls of pickled red cabbage, a couple of pickled chilli peppers and finish with a spoonful of the chilli topping. Mmmm . . . mouth-watering!

> The aubergine will also fry nicely in a non-stick frying pan if you don't have a griddled version.

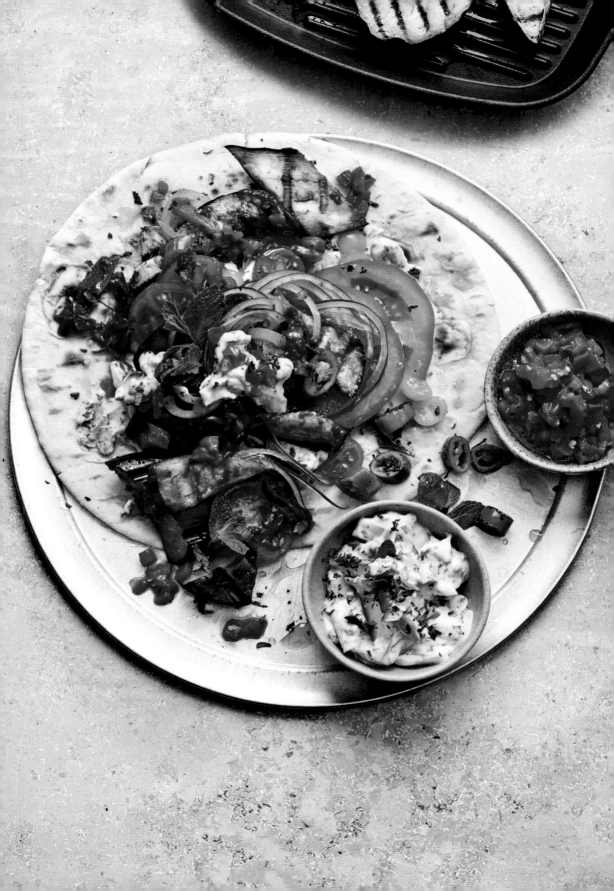

TOFU SAAG PANEER

We're totally in love with this classic veggie Indian dish. Some say it's a side, we say combine it with protein-packed tofu to create a simple, nutritious and delicious dinner.

SERVES 4   **DISH** FRYING PAN   **PREP** 15 MINS + 10 MINS COOLING   **COOK** 40 MINS

600g firm tofu

2 tbsp vegan
  margarine

1 onion

4 garlic cloves

½ a thumb of fresh
  ginger (15g)

1 green chilli

½ tbsp ground cumin

1 tsp ground
  coriander

½ tsp ground
  turmeric

1 tsp fenugreek
  leaves

500g baby spinach

150ml vegan single
  cream, plus extra
  for finishing

1 lemon

4 vegan naans

For the marinade:

2 tbsp nutritional
  yeast

1 tsp ground cumin

salt and pepper

Drain and press the tofu, if necessary. For the marinade, put the juice of half the lemon into a medium mixing bowl along with the remaining marinade ingredients and pinches of salt and pepper.

Cut the tofu into 3cm pieces, then add it straight to the marinade and toss through with your hands. Heat 1 tablespoon of vegan margarine in a frying pan. Once hot, fry the tofu for 15 minutes, turning every few minutes so all sides are golden brown. Meanwhile, peel and chop the onion, garlic and ginger, and slice the chilli, discarding the seeds. Remove the tofu from the pan.

Add the remaining 1 tablespoon of vegan margarine to the pan and fry the onion, garlic, ginger and chilli for 8 minutes. Then add the cumin, coriander, turmeric and fenugreek and fry for 2 minutes. Add the spinach to the pan in stages (as it wilts add a little more), along with 100ml of water. Fry for 10 minutes, or until the spinach has wilted and most of the water has evaporated. Let the mixture cool for 10 minutes, then transfer it to a food processor (see tip below if you don't have a food processor) along with the cream and the juice of the remaining lemon half and process until smooth.

Put the spinach mixture back into the pan, heat it through, and add a few tablespoons extra of water if the mixture is too thick. Taste and season to your liking with salt and pepper, then put the tofu back in.

Finish with a swirl of cream. Heat the naans in a toaster or microwave and serve alongside the curry.

Don't have a food processor? Simply wilt the spinach as instructed, then add the cream and lemon juice directly to the pan.

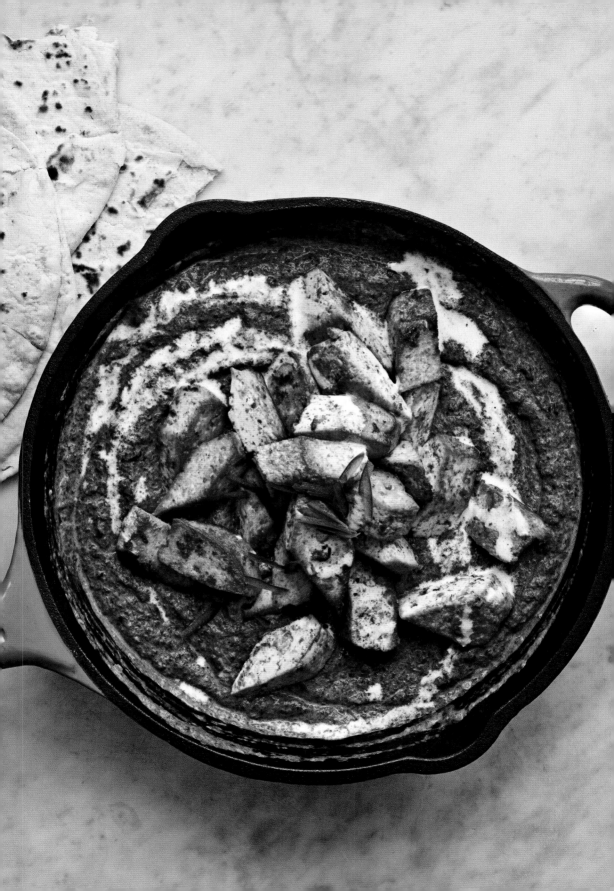

SMOKY SAUSAGE CASSOULET

Picture this. It's cold and miserable outside. You're wrapped up indoors with your hands clutching a large bowl of this outrageously comforting cassoulet. What a life.

SERVES 4   **DISH** OVENPROOF CASSEROLE POT   **PREP** 15 MINS   **COOK** 1 HR 30 MINS

olive oil

8 vegan sausages

1 onion

3 garlic cloves

2 carrots

1 courgette

salt and pepper

2 sprigs of fresh rosemary

2 tsp smoked paprika

3 bay leaves

150ml white wine

2 x 400g tins of butter beans

100g dried apricots

2 x 400g tins of tomatoes

crusty bread, to serve

Put 3 tablespoons of olive oil into an ovenproof casserole pot over a low heat. As soon as the oil is hot, gently fry the sausages on all sides for 10 minutes in total, or until golden and crispy. Fry them in batches, if necessary. Remove the sausages from the pot to a plate and leave to one side.

Meanwhile, peel and chop the onion and garlic. Roughly chop the carrots (keep their nutritious skins on) and the courgette. Add them to the pot, along with ½ teaspoon of salt and a large pinch of pepper, and fry for 10 minutes, adding an extra splash of olive oil if necessary. Pick the rosemary leaves from their stalks, roughly chop them and add to the pot with the smoked paprika and bay leaves. Fry for 3 minutes.

Preheat the oven to 160°C fan/180°C/gas 4. Add the wine to the pan and simmer for 3 minutes, until most of the liquid has evaporated. Drain and rinse the butter beans, and roughly chop the dried apricots. Add them all to the pot with the tinned tomatoes and 100ml of water. Return the sausages to the pot, pushing them down into the liquid. Bring the cassoulet to a simmer, then cover and transfer to the oven for 1 hour, stirring halfway. That's it. Serve with slices of crusty bread for a wonderfully warming meal.

You can sub the sausages with chunky slices of portobello mushroom, added along with the onion.

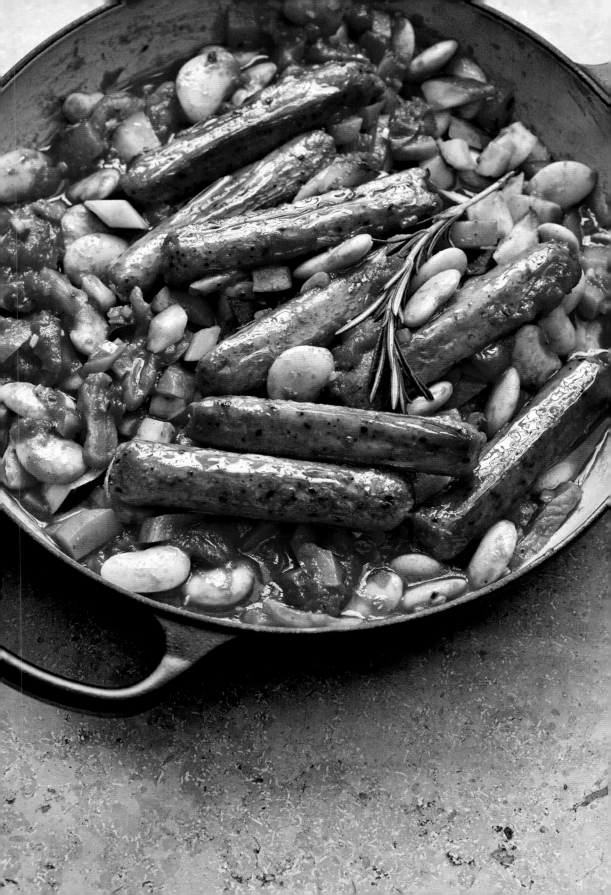

BUTTERNUT SQUASH TAGINE

Ras el hanout, an essential North African medley of spices, deliver the fragrant flavours to this tagine, while the tapenade and soy sauce bring a wonderful depth.

SERVES 4   **DISH** CASSEROLE POT   **PREP** 20 MINS   **COOK** 1 HR 15 MINS

1 red onion

3 garlic cloves

olive oil

4 tomatoes (350g)

1 lemon

1½ tbsp ras el hanout

1 cinnamon stick

salt and pepper

1 medium butternut squash (1kg)

2 x 400g tins of black-eyed beans

50g dried pitted prunes

1 tbsp black olive tapenade

1 tbsp light soy sauce

200g couscous

150g spring greens

a small handful of fresh mint (10g)

a small handful of cashews (30g)

½ a pomegranate

Peel and chop the red onion and garlic. Put 2 tablespoons of olive oil into a casserole pot over a medium heat. Once the oil is hot, fry the onion and garlic for 10 minutes. Meanwhile, roughly chop the tomatoes and zest the lemon. Add the ras el hanout and cinnamon stick to the pot, and fry for 1 minute. Then add the chopped tomatoes, along with the juice and zest of the lemon, large pinches of salt and pepper, and 100ml of water. Give it a stir, then simmer with the lid on for 30 minutes.

Peel the butternut squash, halve it lengthways, scoop out the seeds and chop the flesh into 2cm slices. Drain and rinse the black-eyed beans, and roughly chop the prunes. Add the squash, beans and prunes to the pot, along with the tapenade and soy sauce. Stir, then simmer on a low-medium heat for 30 minutes with the lid on, stirring once halfway through. If the veggies are sticking, add an extra splash of water.

Meanwhile, put the couscous into a mixing bowl and cover with 200ml of hot water from the kettle. Cover with a plate and leave to one side.

Slice the spring greens, discarding any tough ends, and stir them into the tagine. Simmer for 4 minutes with the lid off. Pick the mint leaves off their stalks, roughly chop the cashews and hit the back of the pomegranate half over a bowl to extract the seeds. Top the tagine with the mint leaves, cashews and pomegranate seeds. Fluff the couscous up with a fork, stir in 1 tablespoon of olive oil and pinches of salt and pepper, and serve it alongside the tagine.

> If we can't find black-eyed beans, we'll usually just use whatever tinned beans we have in the cupboard: chickpeas, kidney beans and white beans all work.

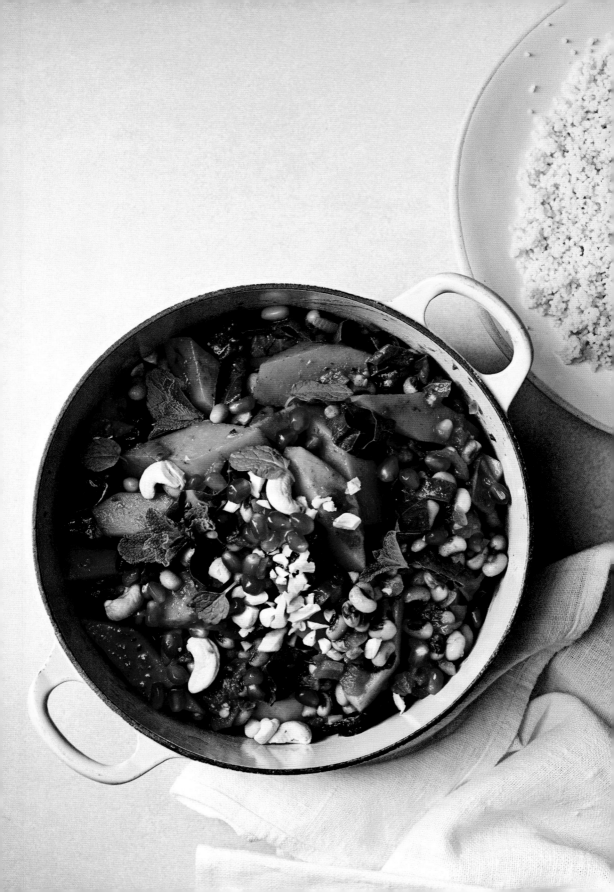

AUBERGINE JALFREZI

The trick to cooking a great jalfrezi is keeping your pan nice and hot. This helps to reduce the stock into a lovely sauce, which wraps around the spicy veggies. Incredible.

SERVES 2   **DISH** FRYING PAN   **PREP** 15 MINS   **COOK** 22 MINS

vegetable oil

2 aubergines (550g)

1 onion

1 tsp cumin seeds

3 garlic cloves

½ a thumb of fresh
   ginger (15g)

1 green pepper

½ tsp chilli powder

1 tsp ground
   coriander

½ tsp ground
   turmeric

1 tbsp tomato purée

400ml vegetable
   stock

1 tsp fenugreek
   leaves

2 tomatoes (180g)

1 red chilli

salt and pepper

a handful of fresh
   coriander (15g)

2 vegan naans

Put 1 tablespoon of vegetable oil into a frying pan on a medium-high heat. Cut the aubergines into 2–3cm pieces, then throw them into the pan and fry for 10 minutes, stirring frequently. Meanwhile, peel the onion and slice thinly.

Remove the aubergines from the pan, then return the pan to the heat and fry the cumin seeds until they start to pop. Add another 1 tablespoon of vegetable oil, throw in the onion and fry for 3 minutes. Meanwhile, peel and slice the garlic and ginger and slice the green pepper, then add them all to the pan and fry for 2 minutes. Add the chilli powder, ground coriander, turmeric and tomato purée and stir for 1 minute, then pour in 200ml of the stock and stir for another minute.

Put the aubergines back into the pan along with the fenugreek leaves and fry for 1 minute. Then pour in the remaining 200ml of stock and stir for 1 minute until the sauce begins to thicken. Quarter the tomatoes, roughly slice the chilli lengthways (keep the seeds if you like it hot), then throw both into the pan along with pinches of salt and pepper and simmer for 1–2 minutes.

Finish with a sprinkling of coriander leaves. Serve with the naans, heated either in the toaster or microwave.

Looking for a protein hit? Slice half a block of tofu into cubes, season generously, coat in cornflour and fry with the aubergines.

SHREDDED 'PORK' + HOMEMADE KIMCHI TACOS

Homemade kimchi and shredded 'pork'. On paper this would require endless hours in the kitchen, but here we rustle up a seriously tasty fusion of flavours in 60 minutes. Result.

MAKES 10 TACOS   **DISH** LARGE ROASTING TRAY   **PREP** 20 MINS   **COOK** 40 MINS

salt and pepper

½ a Chinese cabbage (280g)

500g king oyster mushrooms

vegetable oil

3 tbsp hoisin sauce

2 tbsp soy sauce

1½ tbsp sriracha, plus extra for serving

½ tbsp caster sugar

1 tbsp rice vinegar

½ a thumb of fresh ginger (15g)

½ of a cucumber (150g)

3 spring onions

10 small flour tortillas

sesame seeds

Pour 400ml of hot water from a kettle into a large mixing bowl. Add 1 tablespoon of salt and stir until fully dissolved. Chop the cabbage into 2cm slices and submerge them in the salty water. Leave to one side, stirring occasionally so that the cabbage soaks evenly.

Preheat the oven to 180°C fan/200°C/gas 6 and line a large roasting tray with baking paper. Slice the tops off the king oyster mushrooms, then use your fingers to pull the chunky stalks apart into shreds like shredded 'pork'. Roughly chop the tops, then transfer all the mushroom pieces to the tray, drizzle over 1 tablespoon of vegetable oil, and sprinkle over pinches of salt and pepper. Roast in the oven for 30 minutes. Then stir the hoisin sauce and soy sauce into the shredded mushrooms, and return them to the oven for 10 minutes. Leave the oven on to warm up the tortillas later.

Meanwhile, drain and thoroughly rinse the cabbage under cold water and pat dry with a clean tea towel, then return it to the mixing bowl and add the sriracha, caster sugar and rice vinegar. Peel and grate the ginger into the bowl, and give the kimchi a good mix.

Slice the cucumber into batons and thinly slice the spring onions into strips. When you're ready to serve, quickly pop the tortillas into the oven directly on the shelf for 2 minutes until they've warmed through. Serve the shredded 'pork' alongside the quick homemade kimchi, sliced veggies and warm tortillas, and top your tacos with sesame seeds and extra sriracha, if you like it extra spicy!

Shiitakes with long stalks are also great for shredding into pulled 'pork', in case you're struggling to find king oyster mushrooms.

SRI LANKAN CURRY

Here the coconut milk effectively works as a stock, soaking up all the delicious spices to create a gorgeous sauce for all those lovely veggies.

SERVES 4   **DISH** LARGE ROASTING TRAY   **PREP** 15 MINS   **COOK** 35 MINS

1 butternut squash (1kg)

2 red onions

4 garlic cloves

a thumb of fresh ginger (30g)

600g new potatoes

6 cloves

6 cardamom pods

2 tsp ground coriander

2 tsp ground cumin

2 tsp black mustard seeds

salt and pepper

vegetable oil

2 red chillies

200g tenderstem broccoli

1 x 400g tin of coconut milk

1 lime

a handful of fresh coriander (15g)

Preheat the oven to 200°C fan/220°C/gas 7. Slice the butternut squash in half, spoon out the seeds, peel it, then slice it into 1cm-thick pieces. Peel and roughly slice the onions, peel and slice the garlic and ginger, then put everything into a large roasting tray along with the potatoes. Crush the cloves and cardamom pods in a pestle and mortar (remove and discard the cardamom husks) and sprinkle both over the veggies, along with the ground coriander, cumin, black mustard seeds, ½ teaspoon of salt and a pinch of pepper. Drizzle over 3 tablespoons of vegetable oil, toss with your hands, then roast for 20 minutes.

Slice the chillies (with their seeds), then add them to the tray along with the broccoli and coconut milk. Roast for another 15 minutes.

Cut the lime into wedges, squeeze a few over the curry and decorate with the rest. Finish with a sprinkling of coriander leaves and an extra sprinkling of salt. Make sure you scoop up all the curry-flavoured coconut sauce and drizzle it over the veggies when you serve.

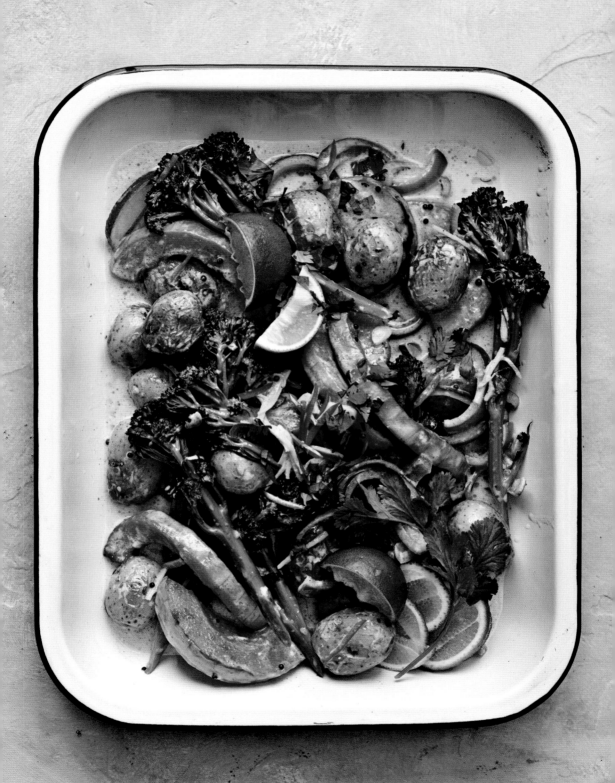

CREAMY FARFALLE

We'll never get bored with blending soaked cashews to create an unbelievably creamy sauce. This is our go-to speedy pasta when we're in a rush and there are hungry people to feed.

SERVES 4   **DISH** LARGE SAUCEPAN   **PREP** 15 MINS   **COOK** 8–12 MINS

150g cashews

400g farfalle

300ml unsweetened plant-based milk

4 tbsp nutritional yeast

½ a lemon

2 tsp soy sauce

1 tsp Dijon mustard

salt and pepper

200g frozen peas

a small handful of fresh curly-leaf parsley (10g)

Put the cashews into a small bowl and cover with hot water straight from the kettle. Leave to one side to soak. Cook the pasta in a large saucepan in salted boiling water as per the packet instructions.

Meanwhile, put the plant-based milk, nutritional yeast, juice from the lemon half, soy sauce, mustard, ½ teaspoon of salt and a large pinch of pepper into a high-powered blender. Don't blend the ingredients yet.

A minute or so before the pasta is ready, scoop out 100ml of the cooking water and pour it into the blender. Add the frozen peas to the pan and cook them through with the pasta for a minute, then drain in a colander.

Drain the cashews and add them to the blender, then blend until smooth. Add extra seasoning, if necessary, then pour the creamy sauce into the pan and heat it through for a minute on a low heat. Put the pasta and peas back into the pan and stir them into the sauce. Roughly chop the parsley and sprinkle on top, along with some freshly ground black pepper. So easy!

Create a nut-free version by skipping the cashews and plant-based milk and using vegan single cream instead.

SUN-DRIED TOMATO PASTA

Black olive tapenade will soon be your new best friend. It brings a welcome saltiness and subtle umami flavour, which blends perfectly with the sweet sun-dried tommies in this pasta.

SERVES 4   **DISH** LARGE SAUCEPAN   **PREP** 10 MINS   **COOK** 10–15 MINS

400g wholemeal fusilli

100g jarred sun-dried tomatoes in oil, drained

2 garlic cloves

½ tsp chilli flakes

2 tbsp capers

3 tbsp black olive tapenade

50g rocket

1 tbsp balsamic vinegar

a handful of fresh basil (15g)

salt and pepper

Cook the pasta as per the packet instructions in lightly salted water in a large saucepan, then drain and reserve 150ml of the cooking water for later.

Meanwhile, drain any excess oil from the sun-dried tomatoes and slice them. Peel and chop the garlic.

As soon as you've drained the pasta, put the pan back on a medium heat and add the sun-dried tomatoes, garlic and chilli flakes. Fry for 2 minutes, adding a splash of oil from the jar of sun-dried tomatoes, if necessary.

Remove the pan from the heat and add the cooked pasta, capers, black olive tapenade, rocket, balsamic vinegar and the cooking water you reserved earlier. Tear in the basil leaves, add a generous pinch of pepper, and give everything a good stir. The pasta shouldn't require any extra salt, but trust your palate and add extra seasoning to taste. Easy.

If you love to meal prep, then you're in the right place! You can make this pasta in big batches for the week. Simply add the basil and rocket on the day to keep it fresh.

PENNE CAPONATA

Vinegar, capers, raisins and olives come together to help create a delicious tomato sauce in this Sicilian-inspired one-pot pasta, where the tender and juicy aubergine steals the limelight.

SERVES 4   **DISH** CASSEROLE POT   **PREP** 15 MINS   **COOK** 30–35 MINS

1 red onion

4 garlic cloves

2 celery sticks

olive oil

½ tsp chilli flakes

salt and pepper

2 aubergines

50g pitted green
    olives

4 tbsp capers

50g raisins

2 tsp dried oregano

4 tbsp red wine
    vinegar

2 x 400g tins of
    chopped tomatoes

400g penne

a large handful of
    fresh flat-leaf
    parsley

a handful of toasted
    almond flakes
    (20g)

Peel and chop the red onion and garlic, and chop the celery into 1cm pieces. Put 2 tablespoons of olive oil into a casserole pot over a medium heat. As soon as the oil is hot, add the onion, garlic, celery, chilli flakes, and large pinches of salt and pepper. Fry for 5 minutes.

Meanwhile, chop the aubergines into 2cm pieces. Add them to the pot and fry for 10 minutes, until they're crispy around the edges. Slice the green olives in half, then add them to the pot along with the capers, raisins and oregano. Fry for 1 minute.

Stir in the red wine vinegar, tinned tomatoes, 700ml of hot water and another pinch of salt and pepper. Next stir in the pasta, bring to the boil, then lower and simmer with the lid on for 10–15 minutes, or until the pasta is al dente.

Meanwhile, pick the parsley leaves off their stalks and roughly chop them. When the pasta is ready, stir in most of the parsley and toasted almond flakes, and season with extra salt and pepper, if necessary. Top with the remaining parsley and almond flakes to serve.

Fresh herbs help to make this pasta sing. Basil and mint will also work if you can't get your hands on fresh parsley.

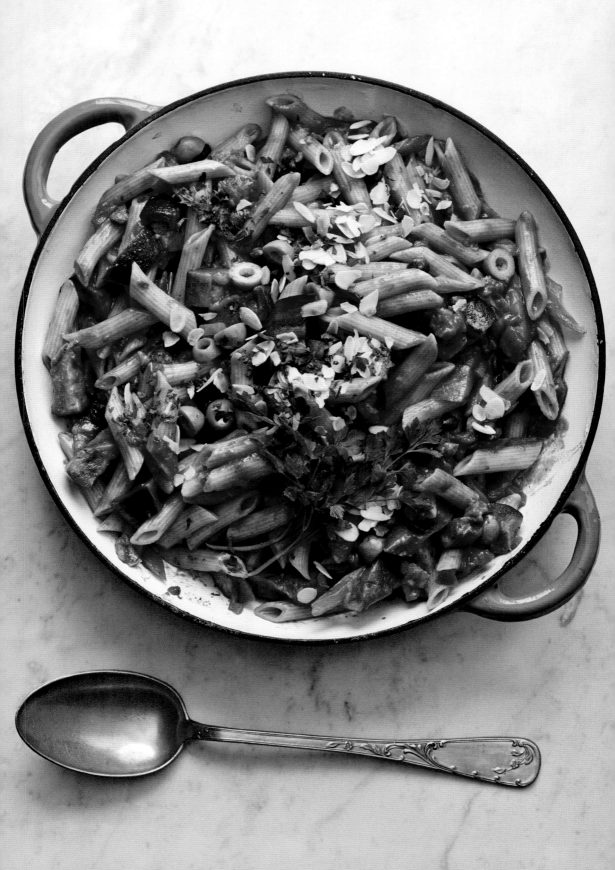

JACKFRUIT BIRYANI

This biryani has a lot to offer. Crispy jackfruit and onions, turmeric-infused rice and spicy cauliflower, all topped with fresh herbs. Oh, and it's all cooked in one tray. Easy.

SERVES 4   **DISH** LARGE ROASTING TRAY   **PREP** 20 MINS   **COOK** 55 MINS

2 x 400g tins of
   jackfruit in brine

3 tbsp Madras
   curry paste

½ tsp ground
   nutmeg

2 onions

vegetable oil

salt

1 small cauliflower
   (450g)

150g green beans

500ml vegetable
   stock

½ tsp ground
   turmeric

300g jasmine rice

50g raisins

Toppings:

8 tbsp vegan plain
   yoghurt (160g)

a handful of fresh
   mint leaves

a handful of fresh
   coriander leaves

Preheat the oven to 200°C fan/220°C/gas 7. Drain and rinse the jackfruit, then cut and thinly slice the inner hard cores, and use a fork to 'pull' the remaining flesh. Put all the jackfruit into a bowl along with 1½ tablespoons of Madras curry paste and the nutmeg and toss until fully coated. Put the jackfruit in one half of a large roasting tray.

Peel and finely slice the onions and put them in the other half of the tray, drizzle with 1 tablespoon of vegetable oil, season with a pinch of salt, then toss and bake for 35 minutes, stirring everything halfway through.

Meanwhile, cut the cauliflower into florets and slice the stalk into bite-size pieces. Top and tail the green beans. Prepare the sauce by combining the veg stock with 1½ tablespoons of curry paste and the turmeric. Rinse and drain the rice.

Remove the tray from the oven, take out the onion and jackfruit and put to one side on a plate. Add the rice, veg stock mixture, cauliflower and green beans to the baking tray. Season with salt, then cover with baking paper or another large tray and bake for 15 minutes.

Pour 100ml of hot water over the rice and put the onion and jackfruit back into the tray, along with the raisins and a small pinch of salt. Bake for 5 minutes, then remove the tray from the oven and top with the yoghurt and the mint and coriander leaves.

> The jackfruit brine and curry paste already add quite a bit of salt, so make sure you taste and season as you go.

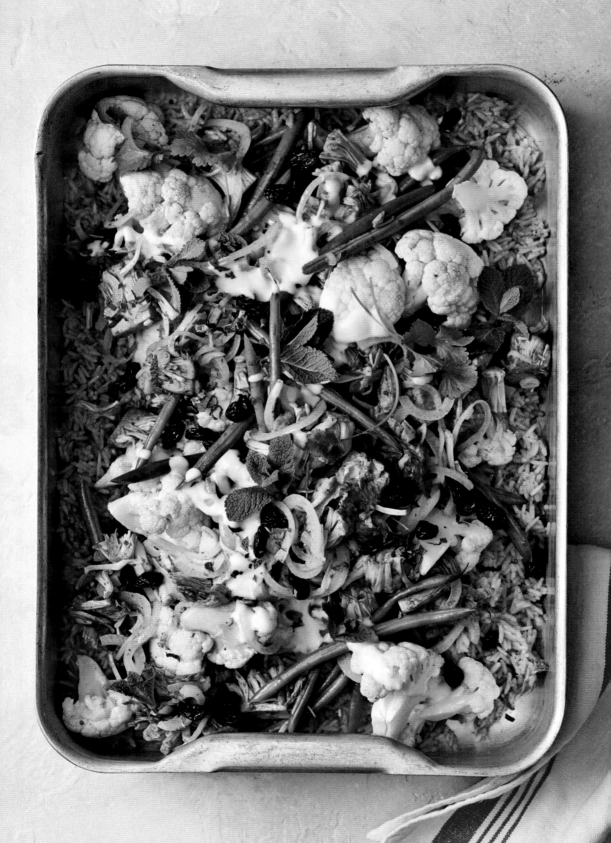

SEAFOOD 'SCALLOP' PAELLA

The OG of one-pot meals. For our paella, we turn to our trusted companion nori – aka seaweed – to deliver that traditional taste of the sea.

SERVES 4   **DISH** SHALLOW CASSEROLE PAN   **PREP** 20 MINS   **COOK** 50 MINS + 5 MINS RESTING TIME

1 onion

olive oil

4 garlic cloves

200g king oyster mushrooms

salt and pepper

1 red pepper

a handful of fresh flat-leaf parsley (15g)

2 tsp smoked paprika

120ml vegan white wine

2 tomatoes (180g)

a large pinch of saffron

500ml vegetable stock

2 tbsp tomato purée

250g paella rice

150g jarred artichoke quarters in oil, drained

1 sheet of nori

100g frozen peas

1 lemon

Peel and chop the onion. Put 2 tablespoons of olive oil into a shallow casserole pan over a medium heat. As soon as the oil is hot, add the onion and fry for 5 minutes. Meanwhile, peel and chop the garlic, and slice the king oyster mushrooms into 1cm-thick circles. Add them to the pan along with a pinch of salt and pepper, then turn the heat up to medium-high and fry them for 10–15 minutes, or until the mushrooms are crispy.

Roughly chop the red pepper. Pick the parsley leaves off their stalks (keep them for later) and finely chop the stalks. Add the red pepper, parsley stalks and smoked paprika to the pan, and fry for 2 minutes. Then add the wine and simmer for 3 minutes, until most of the liquid has evaporated. Meanwhile, roughly chop the tomatoes, then add them to the pan and cook everything for 2 minutes.

Stir the saffron into the stock, then add it to the pan along with 200ml of hot water and the tomato purée. Stir in the rice, bring the paella to a boil, then lower the heat and simmer without stirring for 15 minutes.

Drain any excess oil from the jarred artichokes, then push them down into the paella and simmer for 5 minutes or until the rice is cooked. Add more hot water, if necessary.

Use a pair of scissors to chop the nori sheet into small pieces. When the paella is ready, remove it from the heat and stir in the frozen peas, chopped nori and the juice from half the lemon. Cover the pan with a lid and leave it to sit for 5 minutes. Roughly chop the reserved parsley leaves and slice the remaining lemon half into wedges. Top the paella with the chopped parsley and lemon wedges to serve. Delicious!

> You can substitute the saffron with ½ teaspoon of turmeric, and any mushroom will do if you're struggling to find king oysters.

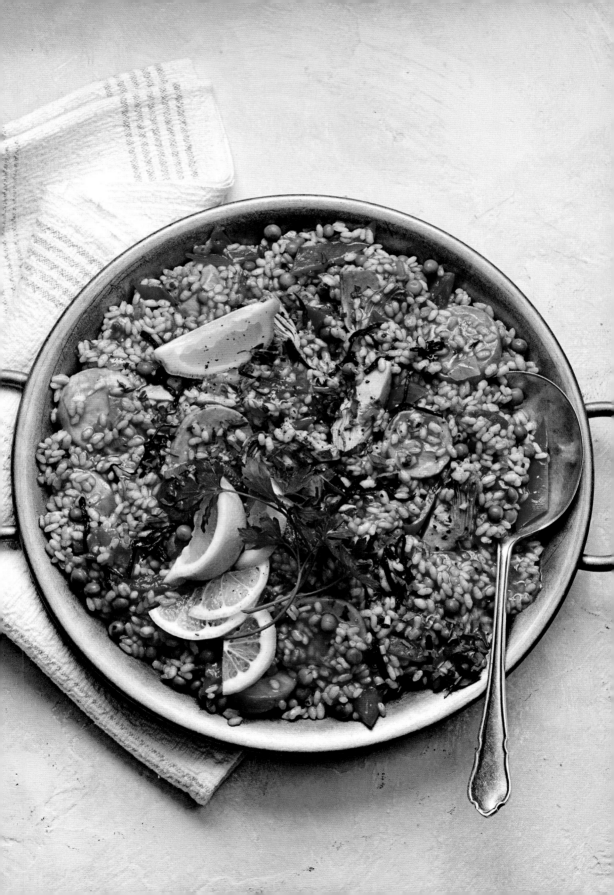

WHOLE ROASTED KATSU CAULIFLOWER

Not many vegetables have the confidence to take centre stage like the cauliflower. Here we roast it in curry spices for that katsu kick and surround it with a creamy stock.

SERVES 4   **DISH** LARGE ROASTING TRAY   **PREP** 30 MINS   **COOK** 45 MINS

1 large cauliflower (1kg)

4 tbsp smooth peanut butter

3 tbsp medium curry powder

3 tsp maple syrup

vegetable oil

salt and pepper

1 onion

4 garlic cloves

3 carrots (300g)

3 celery sticks

500g potatoes

1 tsp garam masala

6 tbsp coconut cream (90g)

500ml vegetable stock

3 tbsp plain flour

40g pecans

1 tbsp dry breadcrumbs

To serve:

2 spring onions

100g radishes

½ of a cucumber (150g)

Preheat the oven to 200°C fan/220°C/gas 7. Trim the leaves off the cauliflower and save them for later. Trim the stalk so the cauliflower stands upright and place in a roasting tray, stalk facing down. In a small bowl, combine 2 tablespoons of peanut butter with 2 tablespoons of curry powder, 1 teaspoon of maple syrup, 2 tablespoons of vegetable oil and a pinch of salt. Rub the mixture all over the cauliflower and roast for 15 minutes.

Meanwhile, peel and finely chop the onion and garlic and dice the carrots, celery and potatoes. Add the veggies to the tray around the cauliflower, drizzle with ½ tablespoon of vegetable oil, and season with pinches of salt and pepper. Roast for 20 minutes.

In a large measuring jug, combine the garam masala with the coconut cream, stock, flour, and the remaining 2 tablespoons of peanut butter, 1 tablespoon of curry powder and 2 teaspoons of maple syrup, along with 100ml of hot water. Prepare the crumb mixture by finely chopping the pecans and combining them with ½ tsp vegetable oil and the breadcrumbs in a small bowl.

Take the tray out of the oven, pour the sauce all over the diced veggies and add the cauliflower leaves from earlier. Finally sprinkle the crumb mixture all over the cauliflower. Roast for 10 minutes.

To decorate, thinly slice the spring onions, radishes and cucumber and spread across the tray.

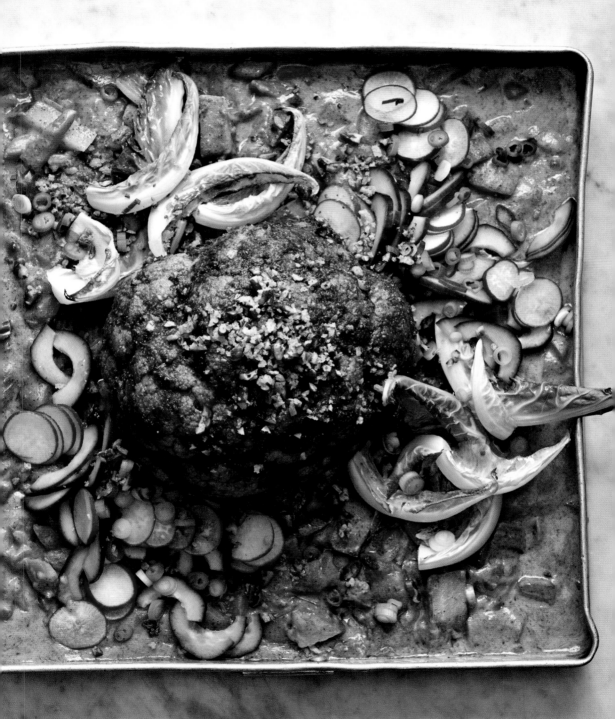

LEFTOVER GREENS FILO TART

We always have leftover greens in the fridge. When we're not blending them in a smoothie, we're scattering them on pastry with a few choice ingredients for an easy meal.

SERVES 4   **DISH** LARGE BAKING TRAY   **PREP** 20 MINS   **COOK** 15 MINS

8 sheets of vegan filo pastry

olive oil

100g sun-dried tomato paste

½ a courgette

2 garlic cloves

salt and pepper

3 handfuls of leftover greens (we use kale, chard and spinach)

1 tbsp pine nuts

For the basil dressing:

a handful of fresh basil (15g)

extra virgin olive oil

½ a lemon

Preheat the oven to 180°C fan/200°C/gas 6. Lay a sheet of filo on a large baking tray and brush with a little olive oil. Add the next sheet of filo directly on top and brush with a little more oil. Repeat with the remaining sheets of filo. Spread the sun-dried tomato paste across the middle. Use a peeler to slice the courgette into ribbons, peel and slice the garlic, and spread both across the filo pastry. Season with salt and pepper and drizzle with olive oil, then scrunch the edges of the filo a little to make a border. Bake for 10 minutes.

Roughly chop the leftover greens and spread over the courgette layer. Sprinkle over the pine nuts and bake for 5 minutes.

Meanwhile, finely chop the basil and put it into a small bowl with 1 tablespoon of extra virgin olive oil and the zest and juice of the lemon half. Stir to combine, then drizzle all over the tart.

Luckily most premade pastry sold in supermarkets, including filo, is now vegan-friendly, but always check the labels.

ROASTED SAGE GNOCCHI

Roasting the gnocchi leaves these golden nuggets crispy on the outside and soft on the inside. Then all you need are a few veggies, fresh sage and a simple dressing. Job done.

SERVES 4   **DISH** LARGE ROASTING TRAY   **PREP** 15 MINS   **COOK** 20 MINS

500g Brussels
   sprouts

1 large broccoli
   (500g)

800g vegan gnocchi

olive oil

salt and pepper

1 small bunch of
   fresh sage (15g)

3 tbsp pine nuts

2 lemons

2 tbsp wholegrain
   mustard

1 tsp maple syrup

extra virgin olive oil

3 large handfuls of
   mixed salad leaves

Preheat the oven to 230°C fan/250°C/gas 10. If your oven doesn't go this hot, get it as hot as you can. Slice off the bottoms of the Brussels sprouts and chop them in half. Slice the broccoli head into small florets and roughly slice the stalk. Put them on a large roasting tray along with the vegan gnocchi, then drizzle over 3 tablespoons of olive oil, and sprinkle over 1 teaspoon of salt and a large pinch of pepper. Give everything a good mix, then bake in the oven for 10 minutes.

Roughly chop the sage leaves, then add them to the tray with the pine nuts. Give everything a good stir and return the tray to the oven for another 10 minutes.

Meanwhile, squeeze the juice from the lemons into a small bowl, then add the wholegrain mustard, maple syrup, 1 tablespoon of extra virgin olive oil, and a pinch of salt and pepper. Stir to combine, then when the gnocchi is ready, stir the dressing and salad leaves into the gnocchi and veggies to serve.

> We love to use this roasted gnocchi as a base, layering it with different veggies and fresh herbs to create new dishes.

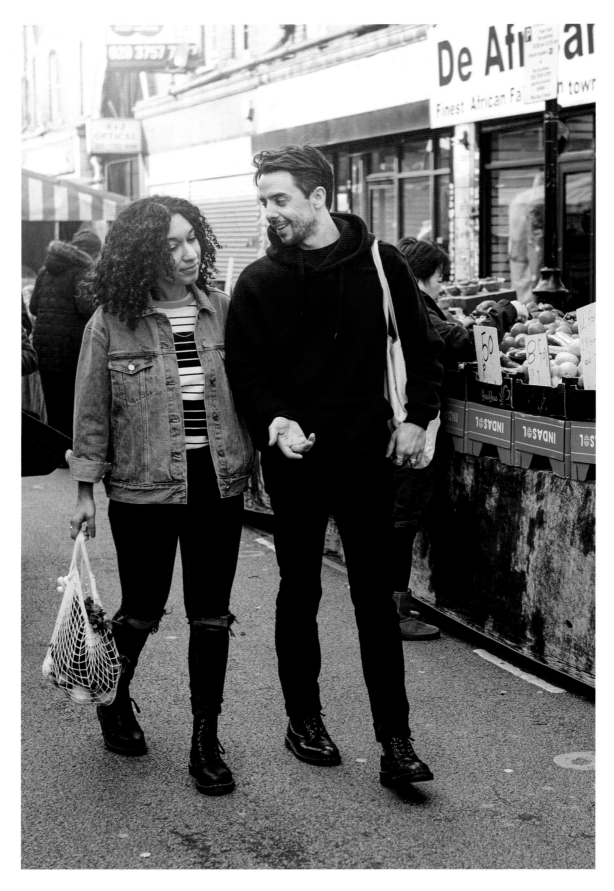

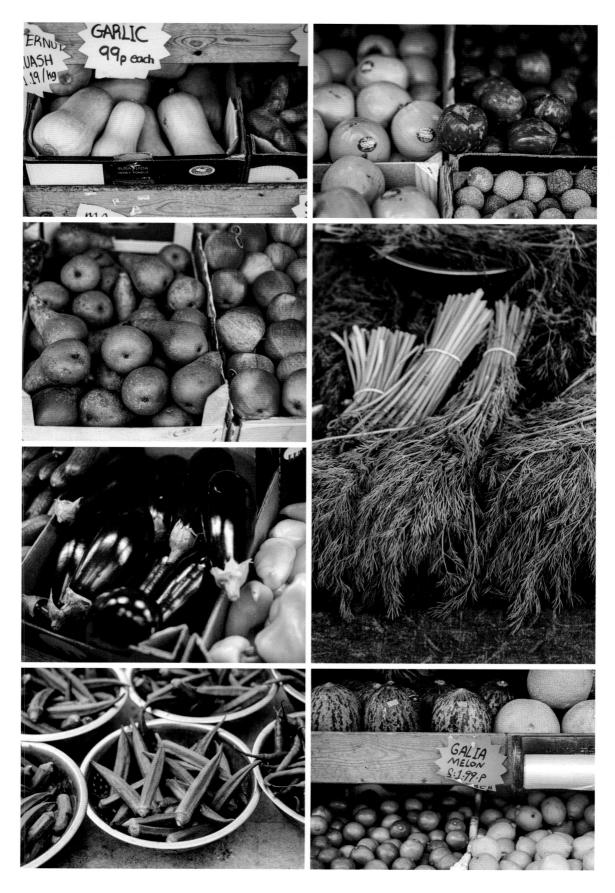

LEEK, POTATO + WHOLEGRAIN MUSTARD PIE

Ben's mum rustles up a mean leek and potato soup. It's a winning flavour combo that works brilliantly in this rustic pie, finished off with a helping of wholegrain mustard.

SERVES 4 **DISH** SHALLOW OVENPROOF CASSEROLE PAN **PREP** 25 MINS **COOK** 1 HR 5 MINS, PLUS 10 MINS COOLING

3 leeks

4 celery sticks

3 carrots

6 garlic cloves

15 fresh sage leaves

olive oil

salt and pepper

1 x 400g tin of cannellini beans

150g frozen peas

250ml vegan single cream

400ml unsweetened plant-based milk

3 tbsp wholegrain mustard

4 tbsp nutritional yeast

1 tbsp plain flour

500g medium potatoes

Slice the leeks and celery, dice the carrots, peel and chop the garlic and roughly chop the sage. Put 2 tablespoons of olive oil into a shallow ovenproof casserole pan on a medium-high heat and once hot, fry the veggies and sage with a pinch of salt and pepper for 20 minutes.

Preheat the oven to 200°C fan/220°C/gas 7. Drain and rinse the cannellini beans and add them to the pan along with the peas, cream, milk, 2 tablespoons of wholegrain mustard, the nutritional yeast, flour and pinches of salt and pepper. Stir until fully combined.

Remove the pie from the heat, then slice the potatoes (skins on) into 3mm-thick pieces and arrange the slices on top to make an even layer. In a small bowl, combine 1 tablespoon of wholegrain mustard with 1 tablespoon of olive oil and pinches of salt and pepper, then spoon it over the top of the pie and spread it over the potatoes. Bake for 45 minutes, until the potato is golden brown and crispy. Leave to cool for 10 minutes before serving.

Nutritional yeast gives this pie a slightly cheesy flavour, which you can also create with a couple of handfuls of grated vegan cheese.

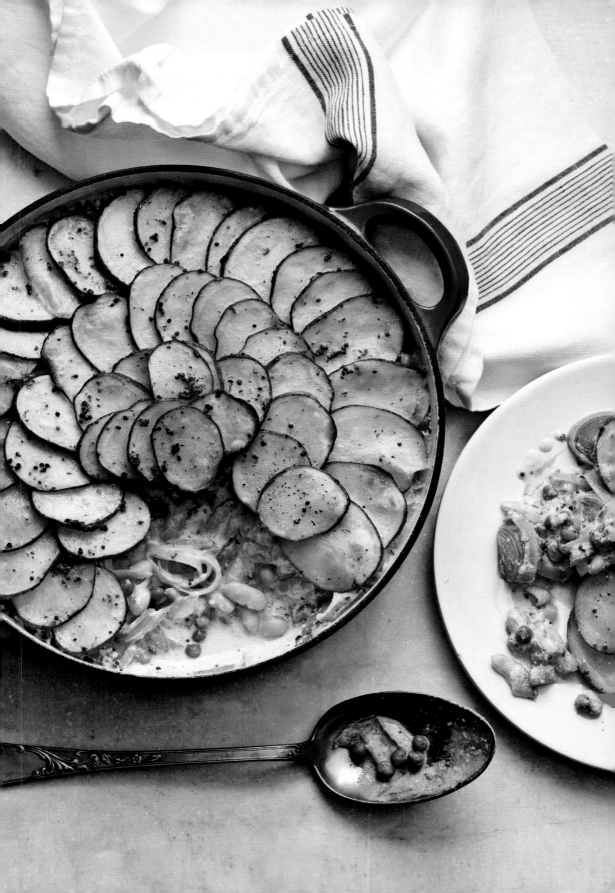

BUTTERNUT SQUASH ORZO

The woody rosemary and fragrant nutmeg work well to bring the best out of the roasted butternut squash, which we combine with orzo, asparagus and grated vegan Parmesan.

SERVES 4   **DISH** LARGE ROASTING TRAY   **PREP** 15 MINS   **COOK** 40 MINS

1 butternut squash

olive oil

salt and pepper

1 tsp ground nutmeg

3 sprigs of fresh
    rosemary

500g orzo

1 litre vegetable
    stock

120g asparagus
    spears

3 tbsp almond flakes,
    plus extra for
    sprinkling

3 tbsp pumpkin
    seeds, plus extra
    for sprinkling

1 lemon

50g vegan Parmesan

Preheat the oven to 180°C fan/200°C/gas 6. Halve, peel and deseed the butternut squash, then cut it into bite-size pieces. Put them on a roasting tray along with 1 tablespoon of olive oil, pinches of salt and pepper, and the nutmeg. Pick the leaves off the rosemary, finely chop and add them to the tray. Toss with your hands to combine, then roast for 15 minutes.

Add the orzo and vegetable stock to the tray, then carefully return it to the oven for 15 minutes.

Add the asparagus, almond flakes and pumpkin seeds and roast for 10 minutes.

To finish, squeeze the juice of the lemon all over and grate most of the vegan Parmesan on top. Stir to combine, then grate over the remaining Parmesan and sprinkle with extra almond flakes and pumpkin seeds.

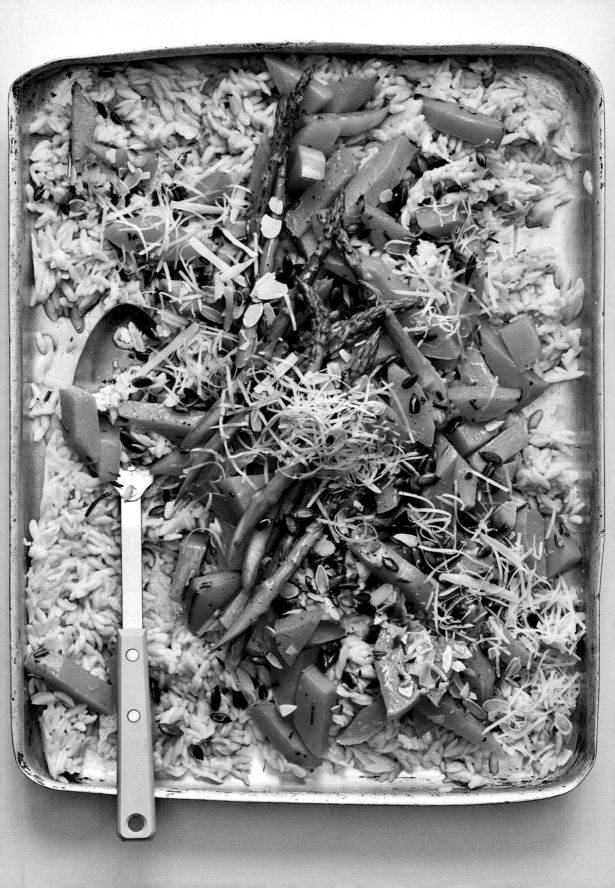

MUSHROOM + ALE FILO PIE

We turn to miso paste in this pie to capture that deep savoury flavour. Mushrooms and lentils create the bulk of the filling, while the light and flaky filo pastry helps to lift the entire dish.

SERVES 4   **DISH** SHALLOW OVENPROOF CASSEROLE PAN   **PREP** 25 MINS   **COOK** 1 HR 20 MINS

8 shallots

olive oil

4 garlic cloves

750g chestnut mushrooms

salt and pepper

2 x 400g tin of brown lentils

2 tbsp brown rice miso paste

2 tbsp tomato purée

4 tbsp apple sauce

2 bay leaves

330ml pale ale

3 tbsp plain flour

3 thick sprigs of fresh thyme

8 sheets of vegan filo pastry

Peel and slice the shallots. Put 2 tablespoons of olive oil into a shallow ovenproof casserole pan on a medium-high heat. Once hot, add the shallots and fry for 6 minutes, stirring frequently until golden. Meanwhile, peel and chop the garlic cloves. Add them to the pan and fry for 2 minutes.

Slice the mushrooms and add them to the pan with a large pinch of salt and pepper. Fry for 20 minutes.

Drain and rinse the lentils and add them to the pan along with the miso paste, tomato purée, apple sauce, bay leaves, pale ale and flour. Pick the leaves off the thyme and throw them in. Give everything a good stir and bring the mixture to the boil, then reduce the heat and simmer for 20 minutes.

Preheat the oven to 180°C fan/200°C/gas 6. Put the sheets of filo on top of the pie one at a time, brushing each sheet with olive oil as you go and rotating the angle of placement each time. Then scrunch the edges of the filo back into the pie and brush the top sheet with a little oil. Bake for 25–30 minutes, or until the filo is golden brown.

> If you want to avoid the pale ale, simply sub with an equal amount of vegetable stock.

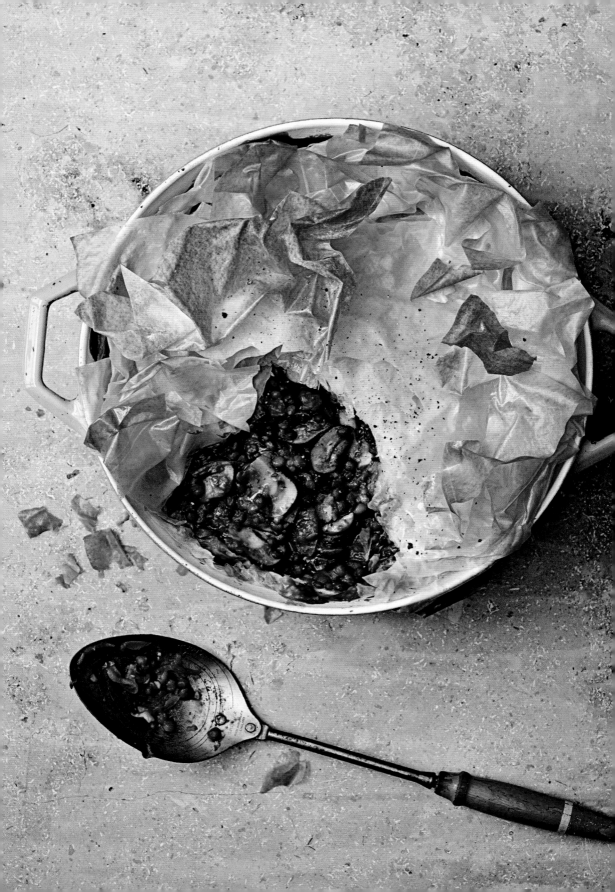

DESSERTS

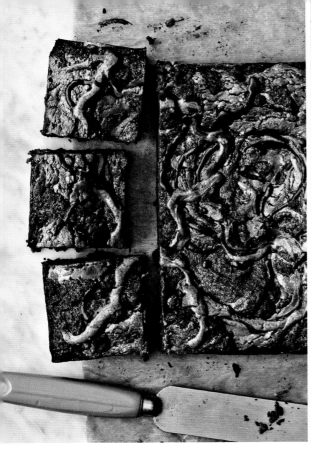

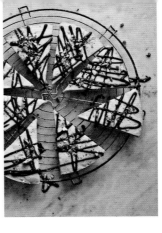

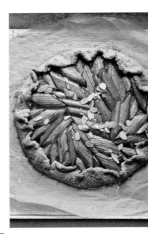

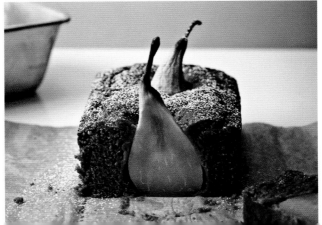

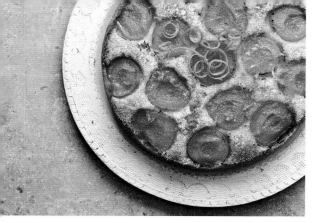

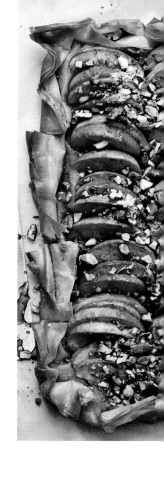

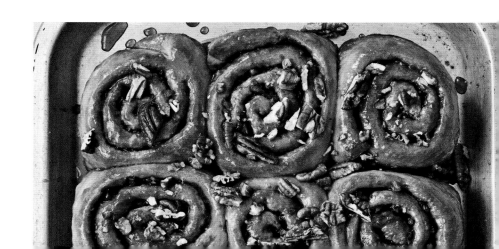

PEANUT BUTTER SWIRL BROWNIES

The ultimate treat. We swirl super-smooth peanut butter into the brownie mixture to create a more gooey texture.

MAKES 9 BROWNIES **DISH** LOOSE-BOTTOMED CAKE TIN **PREP** 20 MINS **COOK** 25–35 MINS

vegan margarine, for greasing

2 tbsp ground flaxseed

60g cocoa powder

150g self-raising flour

250g granulated sugar

salt

110ml vegetable oil

2 tsp vanilla extract

100ml unsweetened plant-based milk

150g vegan dark chocolate

4 tbsp smooth peanut butter

Preheat the oven to 180°C fan/200°C/gas 6. Grease a 20cm loose-bottomed square cake tin with margarine and line with baking paper.

Put the flaxseed into a small bowl, stir in 6 tablespoons of water, then set to one side.

Combine the cocoa powder, flour, sugar and a pinch of salt in a large mixing bowl. Pour the oil, vanilla extract, milk and flaxseed mixture into the dry ingredients and stir until fully combined.

Chop the chocolate into small pieces, add to the brownie batter and give it a good stir. Pour the brownie mixture into the cake tin, then spoon in the peanut butter and use a knife to drag it through the chocolate mixture and create swirl patterns. Bake for 25–35 minutes, or until a toothpick comes out clean.

Remove from the oven and leave to cool for 45 minutes before slicing.

> If you have ground chia seeds at hand, they'll work just as well here as the ground flaxseed.

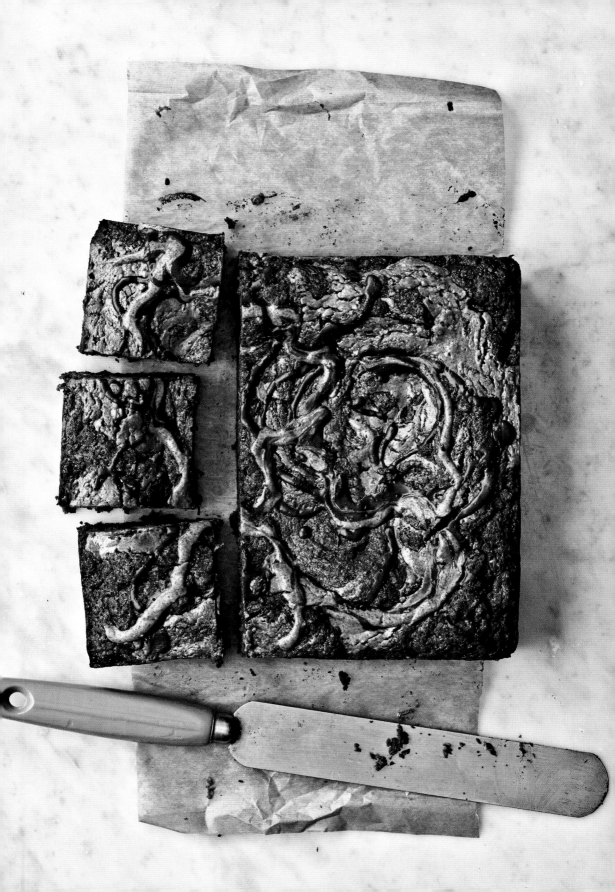

LEMON + POPPY SEED BLONDIES

Roxy was practically raised on poppy seed cake. These blondies are a homage to her proud Polish heritage, and they're mighty delicious, too.

MAKES 9 SQUARES   **DISH** LOOSE-BOTTOMED CAKE TIN   **PREP** 20 MINS, PLUS COOLING   **COOK** 20–25 MINS

100g vegan margarine, plus extra for greasing

180ml soya milk

1 tbsp apple cider vinegar

150g light brown sugar

250g plain flour

1 tsp baking powder

4 tbsp poppy seeds

2 tsp vanilla extract

1 lemon

For the icing:

300g icing sugar

2 lemons

2 tbsp vegan margarine

Preheat the oven to 180°C fan/200°C/gas 6. Grease a 20cm loose-bottomed square cake tin with margarine and line it with baking paper.

Combine the milk and vinegar in a jug to create the vegan buttermilk, and set to one side. Cream the sugar and margarine together in a mixing bowl, then stir in the flour, baking powder and poppy seeds until you have a crumbly mix. Add the buttermilk mixture, vanilla extract and the juice and zest of the lemon, and stir until fully combined.

Pour the blondie mixture into the cake tin and even out with a spatula. Bake for 20–25 minutes, or until a toothpick comes out clean.

Remove the blondies from the oven, run a knife around the edges and leave to cool in the tin for 10 minutes, then turn out on to a rack and leave to cool fully.

For the icing, combine the icing sugar with 3 tablespoons of lemon juice and the margarine until smooth. Once the blondies have completely cooled, spread the icing evenly over them.

Thinly slice the remaining lemon and trim the slices into triangles. Decorate the blondies with the lemon triangles.

If you can wait, pop the blondies into the refrigerator for around an hour so the icing firms up, then cut them into 9 squares.

> Struggling to find poppy seeds? You can either leave them out completely or replace them with sesame seeds.

POLISH BLUEBERRY SPELT CRUMB CAKE

Roxy spent many a summer in Poland on her uncle's blueberry farm, stuffing her face with those tasty purple morsels. This gorgeous crumb cake is another fantastic way to celebrate her roots.

MAKES 9 SQUARES **DISH** LOOSE-BOTTOMED CAKE TIN **PREP** 20 MINS **COOK** 25–35 MINS

220ml soya milk

1 tbsp apple cider vinegar

125g soft light brown sugar

6 tbsp vegan margarine, plus extra for greasing

250g spelt flour

2 tsp baking powder

1 lemon

1 tbsp vanilla extract

450g fresh blueberries

icing sugar, to dust (optional)

For the crumb layer:

80g spelt flour

50g light brown sugar

50g vegan margarine

½ tsp ground allspice

Preheat the oven to 180°C fan/200°C/gas 6. Grease a 20cm loose-bottomed square cake tin with margarine and line with baking paper.

Combine the milk and vinegar in a jug to create the vegan buttermilk and set to one side.

Cream the sugar and margarine together until fully combined, then add the flour, baking powder and the zest of the lemon. Stir until you get a crumb-like consistency. Add the vanilla extract and the vegan buttermilk and stir until fully combined. The mixture will be quite loose.

Pour the cake mixture into the tin and level it out with a spatula. Scatter the blueberries evenly on top.

Put the ingredients for the crumb layer into a small bowl and work the mixture with your fingertips until combined and crumbly. Sprinkle on top of the blueberries and bake for around 25–35 minutes, or until a toothpick comes out clean.

Leave to cool for 15 minutes, then remove from the tin and dust with icing sugar to finish. Cut into 9 squares.

The best thing about this recipe? You can sub the blueberry layer with any berry you like.

APPLE + ORANGE BAKLAVA TART

Our twist on the famous Levantine pastry. Layers of flaky filo, mixed nuts and crunchy apples, all drenched in a sweet orange syrup.

MAKES 6 SQUARES   **DISH** LARGE BAKING TRAY   **PREP** 20 MINS   **COOK** 25–30 MINS

120g nuts
(we use pistachios, almonds and pecans)

1 tbsp caster sugar

3 Pink Lady apples

3 tbsp maple syrup

1 orange

1 tsp ground cinnamon

6 sheets of vegan filo pastry

olive oil, for brushing

vegan vanilla ice cream (optional)

Preheat the oven to 180°C fan/200°C/gas 6. Finely chop the nuts and put them into a small mixing bowl with the sugar. Stir to combine.

Quarter and core the apples, then thinly slice them about 3mm thick. Put the slices into a mixing bowl with the maple syrup, 1 teaspoon of zest and 3 tablespoons of juice from the orange, and the cinnamon. Toss so that the apple slices are evenly coated.

Place a sheet of filo pastry on a large baking tray and brush lightly with olive oil. Place another 2 sheets of filo on top, brushing each sheet with olive oil. Then sprinkle over two-thirds of the nut mixture. Place another 3 sheets of filo on top of the nuts, brushing the sheets with oil as you go.

Arrange the slices of apple on the final sheet of filo, leaving around 2½cm clear on all sides. Save the leftover syrup in the bowl for later. Sprinkle the remaining nut mixture on top, then fold the edges of the filo up over the apples and brush with olive oil. Bake for 25–30 minutes, or until the filo is golden brown and the apples are cooked.

Remove the tart from the oven, pour the reserved syrup all over, and serve with scoops of ice cream.

Simply refrigerate or freeze any leftover filo pastry in an airtight container to save it for another day.

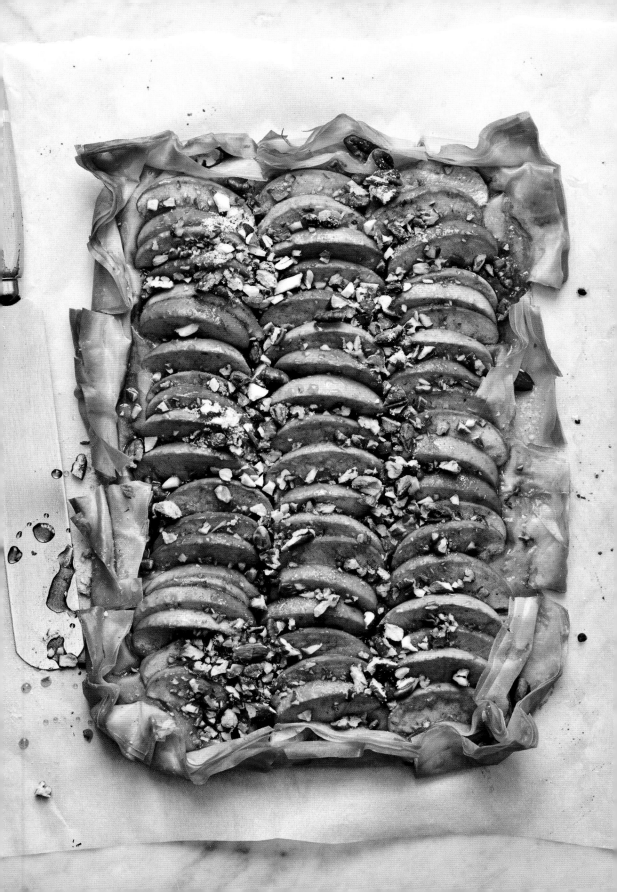

GRILLED FRUITS WITH THYME

Super quick and easy. The lemony and almost minty fresh thyme is the perfect match for these charred fruits.

SERVES 4   **DISH** GRIDDLE PAN   **PREP** 10 MINS   **COOK** 10–12 MINS

1 red grapefruit

4 apricots

2 nectarines

olive oil

5 sprigs of
   fresh thyme

2 tbsp maple syrup

4 cloves

fresh mint leaves

vegan crème fraîche
   (optional)

Slice the grapefruit into 1cm-thick circles. Cut the apricots and nectarines in half, discarding the stones.

Heat a drizzle of olive oil in a griddle pan on a medium-high heat. While the pan heats up, pick the leaves off the thyme and put them into a small bowl along with the maple syrup. Stir to combine.

Place the fruit on the griddle pan and scatter over the cloves. Cook for 5–6 minutes on each side, brushing the maple and thyme drizzle all over. If your pan is small, you may have to do this in two batches.

Serve with a few mint leaves and some vegan crème fraîche, if you like.

Don't fret if you don't have a griddle pan. A non-stick frying pan will do the job nicely.

BANANA SPLIT WITH CHOCOLATE TAHINI

Discovering tahini was an important turning point in our lives. Now we add it to almost anything, including this indulgent twist on a cherished childhood dessert.

SERVES 4   **DISH** FRYING PAN   **PREP** 15 MINS   **COOK** 20 MINS

20g walnuts

20g pecans

2 tbsp vegan margarine

4 firm bananas

6 tsp dark brown sugar

1 tsp ground cinnamon

For the drizzle:

5 tbsp tahini

1 tbsp cocoa powder

2 tbsp oat milk

1 tbsp maple syrup

To serve:

vegan vanilla ice cream

50g vegan-friendly glacé cherries

100g strawberries

Put the walnuts and pecans into a frying pan on a medium heat. Toast for 8–10 minutes, then remove the nuts to a bowl. Wipe out the pan and put it back on the heat.

Melt the margarine in the pan for a few minutes.

Meanwhile, peel the bananas, cut them in half lengthways and sit them cut side up on a chopping board. Sprinkle the banana halves evenly with the sugar and cinnamon. Add the bananas sugar side down to the pan and leave to caramelize for 6–8 minutes. As the caramel bubbles, brush the excess sugar mixture over the tops of the banana halves.

To make the tahini drizzle, whisk the tahini, cocoa powder, milk and maple syrup in a measuring jug. If the sauce is thick, add 1–2 tablespoons of water so that it is thin enough to drizzle, then put to one side. Roughly chop the toasted nuts from earlier and halve the strawberries.

Once the bananas are done, remove the pan from the heat and gently use a fish slice to flip them over so the cut side is facing up.

Top the bananas with scoops of ice cream, the chocolate tahini dressing, the chopped nuts, cherries and strawberries.

Firm bananas are a must. Too soft and they'll fall apart in the pan.

CRUNCHY PECAN + CINNAMON STICKY BUNS

How do we even begin to describe these sticky buns? Well, they're probably the most satisfyingly indulgent things we've ever created. We'll just leave it at that.

MAKES 12 BUNS   **DISH** LARGE OVENDISH   **PREP** 20 MINS + 1½ HRS PROVING   **COOK** 35–40 MINS

650g plain flour, plus extra for dusting

2 tsp fast-action dried yeast

4 tbsp light brown sugar

salt

180ml unsweetened plant-based milk

vegetable oil

For the topping:

60g light muscovado sugar

120g light brown sugar

2 tbsp unsweetened plant-based milk

3 tbsp vegan margarine

80g pecans

For the filling:

4 tbsp vegan margarine

100g light brown sugar

1½ tbsp ground cinnamon

80g pecans

Preheat the oven to 180°C fan/200°C/gas 6.

Combine the flour, yeast, sugar and ½ teaspoon of salt in a large mixing bowl. Measure 180ml of hot water in a jug, then stir in the plant-based milk and pour the lukewarm liquid into the mixing bowl, along with 2 tablespoons of vegetable oil. Combine to form a sticky dough, then transfer to a floured worktop and knead for 2–3 minutes. Add more flour if it's too wet or water if it's too dry. Then grease the inside of the bowl with a small splash of vegetable oil, add the dough and cover with a damp tea towel. Leave to prove in a cupboard or other warm place for an hour, or until it has doubled in size.

For the caramel, put the muscovado sugar, light brown sugar and plant-based milk into a large oven dish. Stir, then break up the vegan margarine and distribute it evenly around the dish. Bake for 10 minutes, stirring halfway through. Then roughly chop the pecans, stir them into the caramel and put the dish to one side to cool down fully. Turn off the oven.

When the dough has finished proving, lightly punch it a few times to remove any air and transfer it to a floured worktop. Roll it out to a rectangle approximately 60cm x 25cm, with one of the longest edges facing you. For the filling, cream together the vegan margarine, light brown sugar and cinnamon in a small bowl, and spread it evenly over the dough, all the way to the edges. Chop the pecans and scatter them evenly on top of the filling. Starting at the long edge nearest to you, roll the dough into a long log by rolling towards the other longest edge. Then use a serrated knife to slice the log at 5cm intervals to create 12 buns. Transfer each bun cut side up to the oven dish, on top of the caramel, and cover with a damp tea towel, leaving to prove for 30 minutes.

Preheat the oven to 180°C fan/200°C/gas 6. Bake the buns for 25–30 minutes, or until they're lovely and golden all over. Let the buns cool down for 2 minutes, then carefully invert on to a large chopping board. It's important you only let the buns cool for a couple of minutes, to avoid the caramel solidifying in the dish. Best enjoyed warm, but they'll also keep for a couple of days!

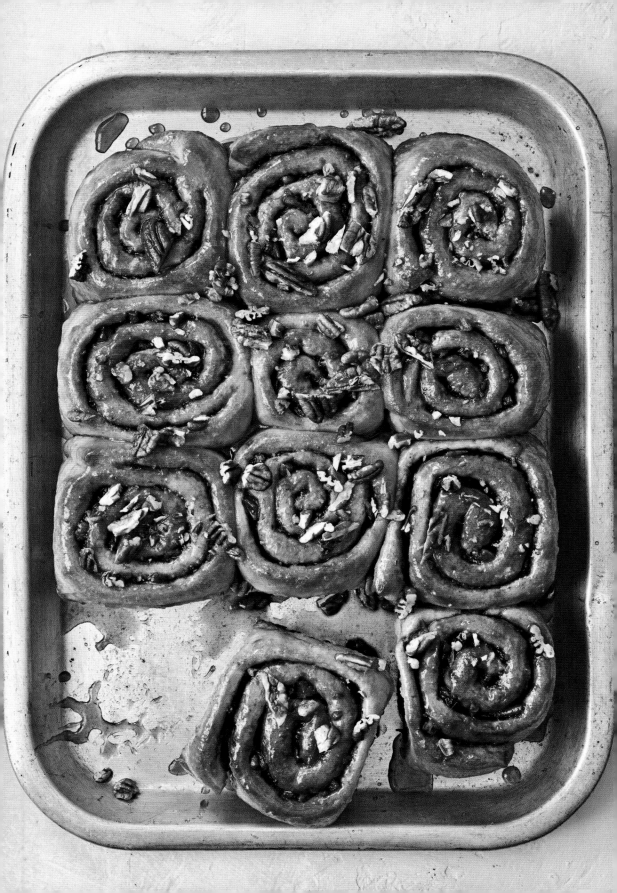

RHUBARB + FRANGIPANE GALETTE

This galette has so much rustic charm it's unreal. The vibrant pink rhubarb, the sweet frangipane and the homemade flaky pastry. Serve with vegan custard for a complete treat.

SERVES 6 SLICES   **DISH** LARGE BAKING TRAY   **PREP** 20 MINS   **COOK** 30–40 MINS

230g plain flour, plus 2 tbsp, plus extra for dusting

40g light brown sugar, plus 6 tbsp

salt

150g vegan margarine, plus 2 tbsp

50g ground almonds

¼ tsp almond extract

2 tbsp aquafaba

400g fresh rhubarb

½ a lemon

a handful of almond flakes

Preheat the oven to 180°C fan/200°C/gas 6. Put the flour, 40g of light brown sugar and a pinch of salt into a mixing bowl. Stir, then rub in 150g of margarine with your fingers until it reaches a crumb-like consistency. If necessary, add 1–2 teaspoons of water so the dough comes together and forms a ball. Wrap the dough in baking paper and pop it into the fridge.

For the frangipane, put the ground almonds into a small mixing bowl along with the almond extract, aquafaba, 2 tablespoons of margarine, 2 tablespoons of light brown sugar and 2 tablespoons of flour. Stir until fully combined. Cut the rhubarb into 5–7cm-long pieces (note: if you want to create a pattern you may need to cut the rhubarb at an angle so that the pieces slot together). Pop the pieces of rhubarb into another mixing bowl, along with 3 tablespoons of light brown sugar and the zest of the half lemon. Toss to combine.

Transfer the dough to the centre of a large sheet of baking paper. Dust a rolling pin and roll the dough into a circle approximately 30cm wide and ½cm thick. Then transfer the dough, still on the baking paper, to a large baking tray. Put the frangipane in the middle of the dough and spread it out into a circle about 25cm wide, leaving 2½cm clear around the edge. Next, arrange the rhubarb pieces on top of the frangipane.

Fold the edges of the pastry over the rhubarb and sprinkle the edges with the remaining tablespoon of sugar. Scatter over a handful of almond flakes.

Bake the galette for 30–40 minutes, or until the pastry is golden. Cover with another tray or loosely with foil after 25 minutes if the almonds are starting to catch.

Remove the galette from the oven. Don't worry if it looks wobbly at this stage, the frangipane will settle as it cools. Leave for 15–20 minutes, until the tart is firm enough to cut.

> Aquafaba? You might be thinking, 'What the . . .?' It's simply the liquid from a tin of chickpeas and it works well as a replacement for egg.

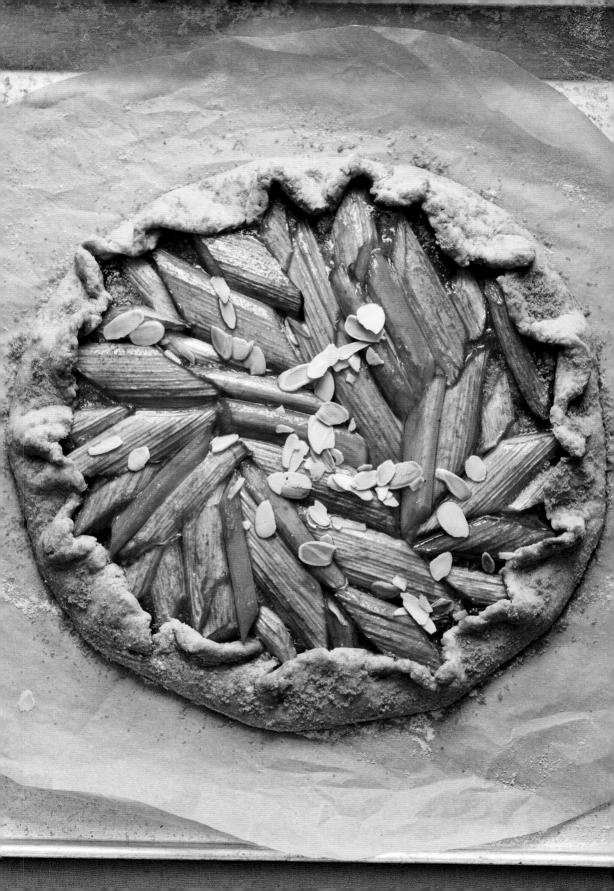

ORANGE + APRICOT UPSIDE DOWN CAKE

We pop our upside down cake back under the grill to caramelize the top. Is it completely necessary? No. But it's well worth the little extra effort.

SERVES 8 SLICES   **DISH** LOOSE-BOTTOMED CAKE TIN   **PREP** 20 MINS   **COOK** 30–45 MINS

120g vegan margarine, plus extra for greasing

1 x 400g tin of apricot halves in syrup

200ml soya milk

1 tbsp apple cider vinegar

150g caster sugar, plus 2 tbsp for topping

100g polenta

200g self-raising flour

½ tsp bicarbonate of soda

1 large orange

2 tsp vanilla extract

Preheat the oven to 180°C fan/200°C/gas 6. Grease a 20cm loose-bottomed round cake tin with margarine and line the base with baking paper.

Drain the apricot halves and arrange them across the base of the cake tin, cut side down.

Combine the soya milk and vinegar together in a bowl and set to one side for a few minutes to create the vegan buttermilk.

Put the sugar and margarine into a mixing bowl and cream together. Add the polenta, flour, bicarbonate of soda, zest from the orange, vanilla extract and the vegan buttermilk. Stir until fully combined, then pour it into the cake tin and bake for 30–40 minutes, or until a toothpick comes out clean. Remove the cake from the oven, run a knife around the edges and leave to cool for 10 minutes. If you want to brown the top, turn the grill on to medium-high and follow the next step, otherwise turn the cake out, apricot side up, and serve as is!

Turn the cake out on to a piece of baking paper and use the paper to drag it back on to the base of the cake tin, still apricot side up. Trim the excess baking paper closely around the cake so it doesn't catch under the grill. Sprinkle the top of the cake with 2 tablespoons of sugar, then pop it under the grill for 2–5 minutes, or until golden brown and slightly charred. Keep an eye on it to make sure it doesn't burn.

> You can always use fresh apricots when they're in season – use 8 ripe but firm apricots, halved and stones removed.

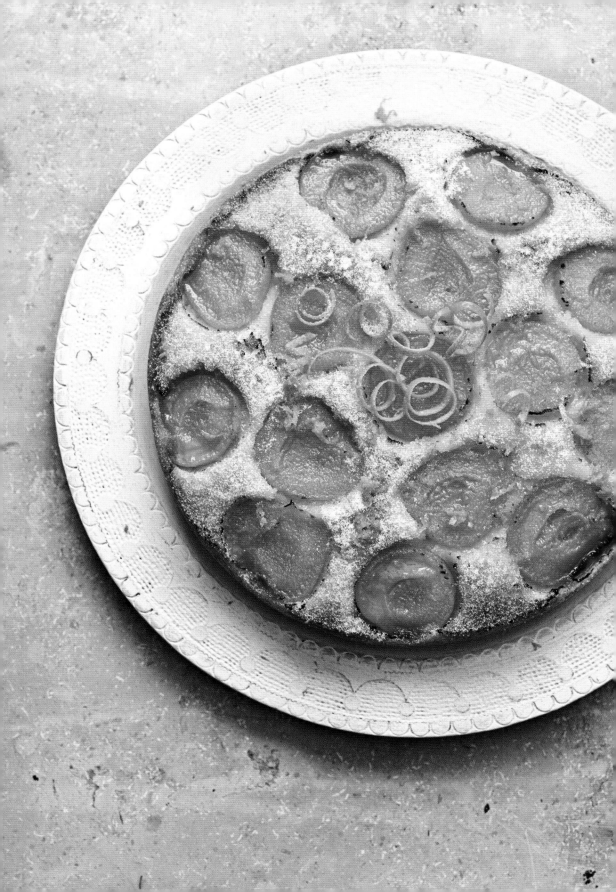

BOOZY CARIBBEAN PEAR CAKE

Our spin on a classic Caribbean cake. Fresh pears take pride of place alongside cinnamon, ginger, nutmeg – and of course rum – to create a wonderfully rich treat.

SERVES 9 SLICES **DISH** LARGE LOAF TIN **PREP** 15 MINS **COOK** 40–50 MINS

100g vegan
margarine, plus
extra for greasing

80g dark brown
sugar

4 tbsp treacle

4 tbsp golden syrup

1 tsp vanilla extract

140ml dark rum

1 tbsp apple cider
vinegar

200g self-raising
flour

4 tsp ground ginger

1 tsp ground
cinnamon

½ tsp ground nutmeg

2 medium ripe
Conference pears

icing sugar,
for dusting

Preheat the oven to 180°C fan/200°C/gas 6. Grease a large loaf tin with margarine and line with baking paper.

Cream the margarine and sugar together in a large mixing bowl. Add the treacle, golden syrup and vanilla extract and stir to combine. Pour in the rum and vinegar and give everything a stir. Add the flour, ginger, cinnamon and nutmeg, and stir until everything is fully combined. Pour the cake mixture into the loaf tin.

Peel the pears, trim their bottoms so they have a flat base, and place them upright in the loaf tin, pushing them down gently into the cake mixture. Bake for 40–50 minutes, or until a toothpick comes out clean and the pears are soft.

Remove the cake from the oven and leave to cool in the tin for a few minutes. Then take it out of the tin and place on a rack. Once fully cooled, dust with icing sugar to decorate.

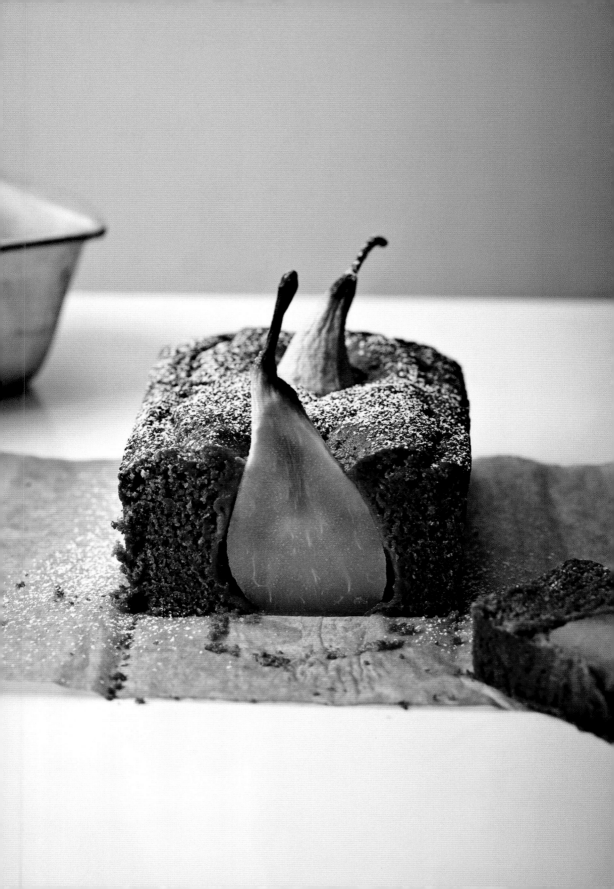

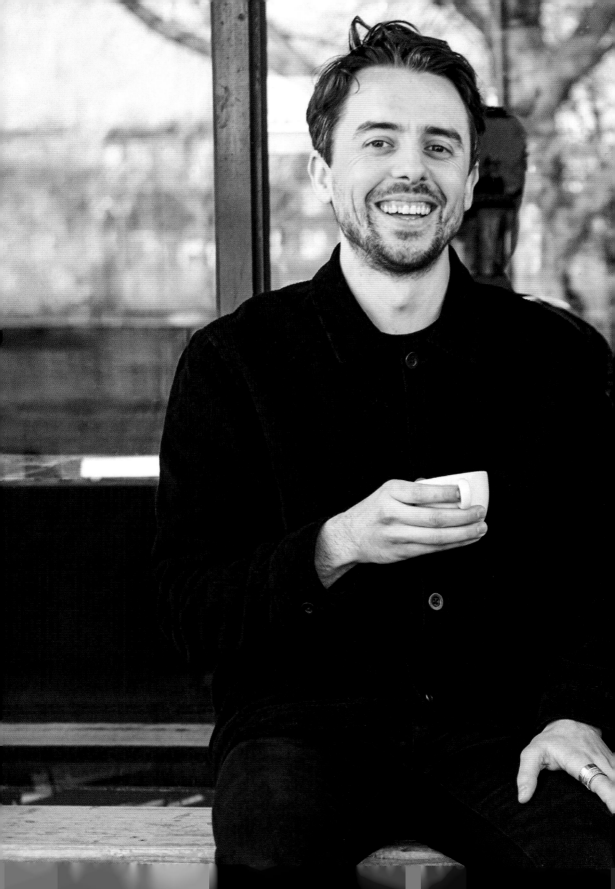

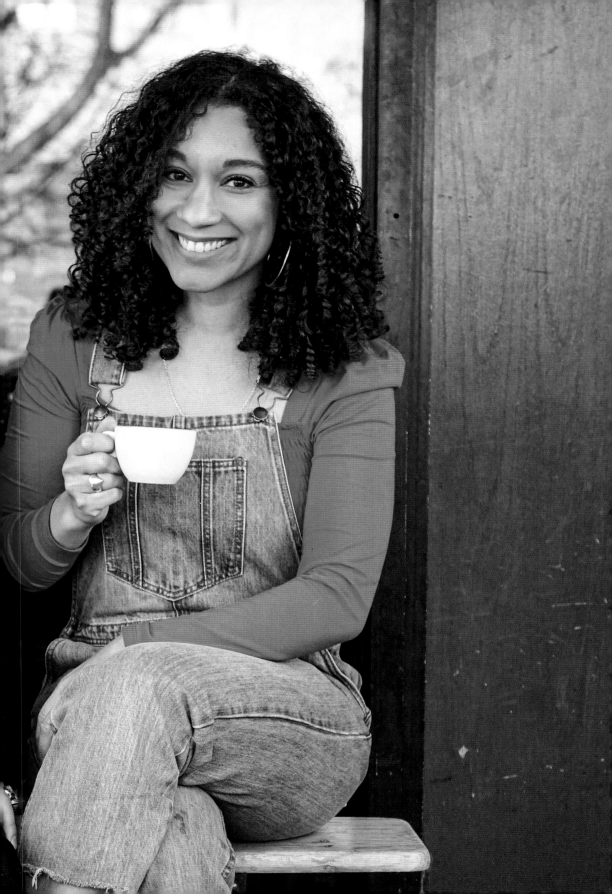

CARDAMOM + PISTACHIO SHORTBREAD

These light and flaky shortbread biscuits use icing sugar for a softer texture, while the cardamom and pistachios complement each other like two best friends.

MAKES 8 TRIANGLES　**DISH** LOOSE-BOTTOMED CAKE TIN　**PREP** 15 MINS　**COOK** 30 MINS

160g vegan margarine, plus extra for greasing

80g icing sugar

1 tsp vanilla extract

salt

6 cardamom pods

250g plain flour

To decorate:

80g icing sugar

1 tbsp cocoa powder

a small handful of pistachios

Preheat the oven to 160°C fan/180°C/gas 4. Grease a 20cm loose-bottomed round cake tin with margarine and line the base with baking paper.

In a mixing bowl, cream together the margarine, icing sugar, vanilla extract and a pinch of salt. Crush the cardamom pods in a pestle and mortar. Remove the pods and grind the seeds until fine, then add to the mixing bowl along with the flour and stir to combine.

Transfer the mixture to the cake tin, smooth it out and prick with a fork a few times. Bake for 30 minutes.

Leave to cool for a couple of minutes in the tin, then carefully remove. Cut the shortbread into triangles on a chopping board, then transfer to a rack to fully cool.

To make the icing, combine the icing sugar with the cocoa powder and 3½ teaspoons of water and stir until smooth (add a little more water if it's too thick).

Once the shortbread triangles have fully cooled, use a spoon to drizzle the icing over them. Peel and roughly chop the pistachios then sprinkle on top.

> If you're not a huge fan of cardamom, 1 teaspoon of ground ginger would work just as well.

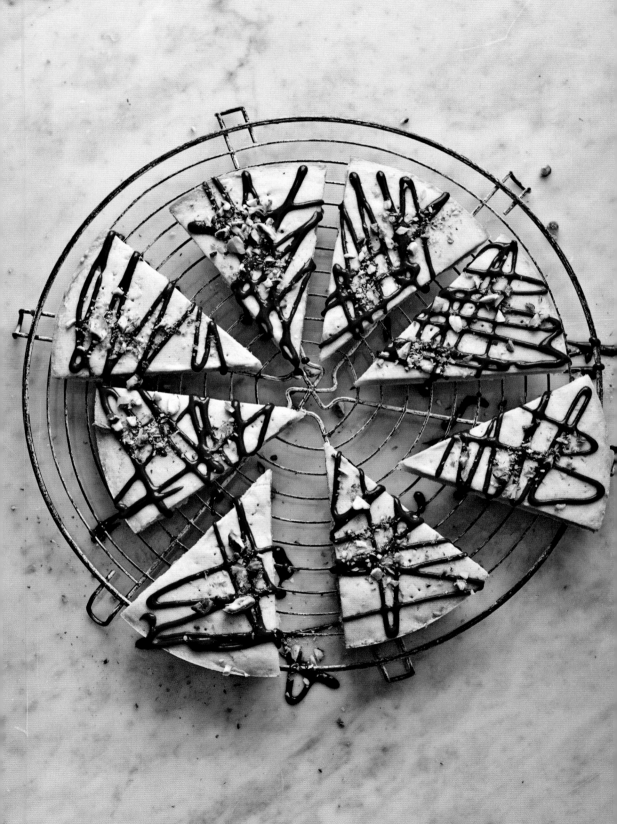

THANKS

This book is a melting pot (pun intended, ahem) of so many things we've learned over the past few years. This is precisely how we love to cook, especially when we're busy and tired. We're talking about quick and easy one-pot cooking that delivers on the most important thing... flavour. It's honestly a privilege to share our tasty creations with the world so we want to say a humongous thank you to everyone who has made this book possible.

Firstly, where would we be without our community? A big worldwide thank you to everyone who has bought this book, follows us on social media, watches our videos or recreates our recipes at home. We are forever grateful for your support and we couldn't have done this without you. So Vegan has been an unforgettable adventure so far and we are beyond excited to be on this journey with all of you.

To our amazing editor, Ione. Where do we start? We are still pinching ourselves that this is really happening! You have steered the ship brilliantly and you have helped shape this book into something we can all be incredibly proud of. Thank you for believing in So Vegan and welcoming us into the Michael Joseph family.

To Sarah for designing this beautiful book, as well as Emma, Liv, Jen, Claire, Gail, Rebecca, Agatha, Vicky and the entire team at MJ, you're all absolutely brilliant and we couldn't have asked for a better team.

A huge thank you to Ariella, Molly and everyone at United Agents for your continued support and commitment to So Vegan.

To our wonderful cookbook crew: Dan for all the gorgeous photos, Bianca for styling the stunning recipes, and, of course, a big thank you to Linda, Janet, Aloha, India and Jake. You're all stars.

Thank you to Katy and Annie for looking through every single recipe with a fine toothcomb! You are both terrific. To Anita for working your magic and calculating all the nutritional values for each recipe, thank you!

Big love to our wonderful freelance team; Rebecca, Jess (aka The Crude Vegan) and Jake. You're a talented bunch who often put us to shame and it's a privilege working with you.

Thank you to our manager Chloe for being a constant voice of reason. And to Adam, Nhikil and Ashley for all your worldly and business advice. You constantly inspire us to work harder and achieve our ambitions.

A big shout out to Plant Based News, Made In Hackney, Vevolution and Veganuary, and everyone else in the vegan community that we're super proud to be a part of. Thanks for fighting the good fight.

And lots of love to our favourite locals for allowing us to take photos at their locations for this book: Fowlds Cafe for serving up delicious caffeinated beverages and Oli Food Centre for being the best Turkish supermarket there is!

And last but by no means least, thank you to our friends and family who put up with us talking about So Vegan literally all the time. Your daily encouragement motivates us and keeps us going when we need it the most. We feel so lucky to have every single one of you. Oh, and, of course, thank you to the one and only Bento for all the cuddles.

Roxy + Ben

NUTRITIONAL INFORMATION

	PER SERVING	PROTEIN	FAT	CARBS	FIBRE
ROASTED BEETROOT + ORANGE SALAD	604 cals (for 4)	12g	21g (2g saturates)	87g (58g total sugars)	13g
TANGY ROASTED FENNEL + BULGUR SALAD	580 cals	16g	28g (3g saturates)	58g (12g total sugars)	15g
FIERY CHIPOTLE FRITTERS Per serving (fritter) (without avocado and creme)	116 cals	4g	4g (1g saturates)	8g (2g total sugars)	2g
SPRING GREEN SALAD	481cals	17g	20g (3g saturates)	54g (10g total sugars)	12g
OUR GO-TO RAMEN	505 cals	21g	21g (2g saturates)	50g (9g total sugars)	15g
LOADED SWEET POTATO WEDGES	660 cals (for 4)	17g	21g (4g saturates)	89g (29g total sugars)	21g
RAINBOW NOODLES	626 cals	17g	24g (4g saturates)	78g (36g total sugars)	12g
ROASTED PARSNIP + CRISPY PITTA FATTOUSH	431 cals	11g	17g (2g saturates)	52g (15g total sugars)	14g
BLACK DHAL (including 4 x 150g naan breads)	906 cals	42g	18g (4g saturates)	134g (17g total sugars)	19g
BLACK DHAL (without naan breads)	492 cals	28g	12g (2g saturates)	60g (13g total sugars)	15g
TRAYBAKE MUJADARA + PARSLEY SALAD	443 cals (without additional olive oil)	16g	10g (1g saturates)	67g (13g total sugars)	12g
CRUNCHY ASIAN SALAD WITH GINGER DRESSING	390 cals	12g	28g (5g saturates)	17g (12g total sugars)	9g
MINI GARDEN FLATBREADS	520 cals	20g	8g (1g saturates)	86g (10g total sugars)	13g
SWEET POTATO HASH WITH SCRAMBLED HARISSA TOFU	563 cals	19g	28g (5g saturates)	52g (20g total sugars)	14g
BALSAMIC BRUSSELS SPROUT SALAD	286 cals	8g	17g (3g saturates)	21g (18g total sugars)	11g

	PER SERVING	PROTEIN	FAT	CARBS	FIBRE
NO-WASTE HARISSA CAULIFLOWER	484 cals	21g	21g (2g saturates)	44g (17g total sugars)	16g
ROCKET HASSELBACK POTATOES	716 cals	24g	29g (3g saturates)	80g (7g total sugars)	19g
3 BEANS + CHICORY SALAD	499 cals	21g	22g (4g saturates)	48g (4g total sugars)	10g
ROASTED VEGETABLE MEZZE	390 cals (for 4)	14g	11g (2g saturates)	54g (15g total sugars)	12g
MEXICAN QUINOA SALAD	336 cals	14g	9g (1g saturates)	45g (10g total sugars)	10g
CAJUN MESS WITH CRUNCHY TORTILLA CRISPS	716 cals	21g	36g (8g saturates)	68g (17g total sugars)	20g
FARRO, KALE + COCONUT SALAD	557 cals	14g	32g (12g saturates)	51g (8g total sugars)	6g
ROASTED POTATO ALLA NORMA	458 cals	9g	17g (6g saturates)	61g (12g total sugars)	12g
WEEKNIGHT PEANUT BUTTER UDON	524 cals	18g	25g (4g saturates)	50g (22g total sugars)	13g
BROCCOLI, LEEK + CHUTNEY TART	482 cals	8g	33g (18g saturates)	36g (8g total sugars)	5g
PEARL BARLEY CHILLI	470 cals	17g	7g (2g saturates)	77g (18g total sugars)	14g
MUSHROOM TIKKA MASALA	541 cals	19g	13g (3g saturates)	83g (12g total sugars)	7g
WILD MUSHROOM + ASPARAGUS RISOTTO	509 cals	11g	10g (3g saturates)	80g (5g total sugars)	5g
SHIITAKE LAKSA	433 cals	21g	23g (8g saturates)	32g (11g total sugars)	8g
SEASIDE TOFISH GOUJONS + CHIPS	644 cals	23g	29g (4g saturates)	66g (9g total sugars)	12g

	PER SERVING	PROTEIN	FAT	CARBS	FIBRE
CREAMY CAULIFLOWER KORMA (without naans and toppings etc)	453 cals	11g	26g (3g saturates)	39g (18g total sugars)	9g
CREAMY CAULIFLOWER KORMA (with naans and toppings)	925 cals	26g	36g (5g saturates)	118g (26g total sugars)	13g
ALOO GOBI TRAYBAKE	445 cals	14g	12g (4g saturates)	65g (16g total sugars)	12g
SUPER GREEN GNOCCHI	482 cals	16g	16g (3g saturates)	65g (4g total sugars)	11g
MEDITERRANEAN ORZO	659 cals	22g	13g (2g saturates)	107g (17g total sugars)	15g
TOFU 'BACON' CAESAR SALAD	508 cals	26g	33g (6g saturates)	23g (8g total sugars)	8g
LEMONY LINGUINE	574 cals	19g	17g (3g saturates)	81g (9g total sugars)	11g
CHEEKY CHIMICHURRI FAJITAS	227 cals (per fajita if serving 8)	6g	10g (2g saturates)	26g (5g total sugars)	5g
CHEAT'S PIZZA	498 cals (for 4)	6g	35g (18g saturates)	37g (8g total sugars)	4g
CHICKPEA KOFTE KEBABS	580 cals	20g	29g (4g saturates)	56g (5g total sugars)	11g
TOFU SATAY WITH CAULIFLOWER RICE	358 cals	24g	20g (5g saturates)	18g (13g total sugars)	6g
SWEET POTATO THAI GREEN CURRY	481 cals	7g	22g (18g saturates)	58g (17g total sugars)	10g
ROASTED SQUASH, CAULIFLOWER + SAGE	541 cals	19g	26g (3g saturates)	49g (26g total sugars)	17g
AUBERGINE + COURGETTE BAKE	212 cals	7g	10g (2g saturates)	19g (14g total sugars)	7g
CARIBBEAN FEAST	803 cals	18g	37g (17g saturates)	93g (19g total sugars)	13g

	PER SERVING	PROTEIN	FAT	CARBS	FIBRE
SWEET + SOUR JACKFRUIT FAKEAWAY	763 cals	13g	9g (1g saturates)	148g (69g total sugars)	18g
'FISHCAKES' WITH HOMEMADE SLAW + MAYO	382 cals	18g	16g (1g saturates)	34g (6g total sugars)	15g
COURGETTE CANNELLONI WITH TOFU RICOTTA (without bread)	352 cals	20g	22g (3g saturates)	15g (11g total sugars)	6g
'CHICKEN' SUPREME	276 cals	8g	14g (2g saturates)	18g (6g total sugars)	4g
HARISSA-SPICED AUBERGINE (including 1 tbsp soya yogurt per serving)	340 cals	17g	13g (1g saturates)	32g (13g total sugars)	15g
LAZY LASAGNE	631 cals (for 4)	16g	30g (8g saturates)	57g (15g total sugars)	8g
ALMOND + CHICKPEA CURRY (without naans, for 4)	507 cals	16g	32g (19g saturates)	34g (12g total sugars)	11g
MUSHROOM STROGANOFF	557 cals	19g	15g (2g saturates)	82g (10g total sugars)	9g
AUBERGINE KEBABS WITH TZATZIKI + CHILLI (with 1 x 60g flatbread)	311 cals	11g	9g (1g saturates)	44g (14g total sugars)	8g
TOFU SAAG PANEER	695 cals	37g	23g (4g saturates)	82g (8g total sugars)	7g
SMOKY SAUSAGE CASSOULET	611 cals	19g	22g (2g saturates)	68g (26g total sugars)	22g
BUTTERNUT SQUASH TAGINE	606 cals	22g	13g (2g saturates)	93g (24g total sugars)	17g
AUBERGINE JALFREZI	656 cals	19g	20g (3g saturates)	93g (21g total sugars)	16g
SHREDDED 'PORK' + HOMEMADE KIMCHI TACOS	116 cals	4g	3g (1g saturates)	18g (5g total sugars)	2g
CREAMY FARFALLE	669 cals	28g	21g (4g saturates)	86g (8g total sugars)	11g

	PER SERVING	PROTEIN	FAT	CARBS	FIBRE
SRI LANKAN CURRY	509 cals	10g	26g (15g saturates)	53g (20g total sugars)	12g
SUN-DRIED TOMATO PASTA	441 cals	16g	7g (1g saturates)	72g (8g total sugars)	15g
PENNE CAPONATA	592 cals	19g	12g (2g saturates)	95g (23g total sugars)	14g
JACKFRUIT BIRYANI	619 cals	15g	10g (1g saturates)	110g (40g total sugars)	16g
SEAFOOD 'SCALLOP' PAELLA	410 cals	10g	9g (1g saturates)	63g (9g total sugars)	8g
WHOLE ROASTED KATSU CAULIFLOWER	632 cals	18g	30g (8g saturates)	64g (23g total sugars)	18g
LEFTOVER GREENS FILO TART	394 cals	7g	26g (3g saturates)	31g (4g total sugars)	5g
ROASTED SAGE GNOCCHI	626 cals	20g	25g (4g saturates)	72g (9g total sugars)	19g
LEEK, POTATO + WHOLEGRAIN MUSTARD PIE	480cals	20g	17g (2g saturates)	53g (14g total sugars)	19g
BUTTERNUT SQUASH ORZO	764 cals	26g	19g (4g saturates)	116g (14g total sugars)	14g
MUSHROOM + ALE FILO PIE	523 cals	20g	16g (2g saturates)	63g (9g total sugars)	14g
PEANUT BUTTER SWIRL BROWNIES	426 cals	7g	20g (5g saturates)	52g (38g total sugars)	4g
LEMON + POPPY SEED BLONDIES	397 cals	5g	10g (2g saturates)	71g (49g total sugars)	1g
POLISH BLUEBERRY SPELT CRUMB CAKE	311 cals	6g	10g (2g saturates)	48g (24g total sugars)	3g
APPLE + ORANGE BAKLAVA TART	287cals	8g	8g (2g saturates)	28g (14g total sugars)	3g

	PER SERVING	PROTEIN	FAT	CARBS	FIBRE
GRILLED FRUITS WITH THYME	105 cals	2g	3g (0g saturates)	17g (17g total sugars)	3g
BANANA SPLIT WITH CHOCOLATE TAHINI (without ice cream)	417 cals	8g	23g (4g saturates)	41g (29g total sugars)	6g
CRUNCHY PECAN + CINNAMON STICKY BUNS	469 cals	7g	17g (2g saturates)	70g (28g total sugars)	3g
RHUBARB + FRANGIPANE GALETTE	396 cals	7g	21g (4g saturates)	43g (22g total sugars)	3g
ORANGE + APRICOT UPSIDE DOWN CAKE	326 cals	4g	10g (2g saturates)	55g (26g total sugars)	2g
BOOZY CARIBBEAN PEAR CAKE	260 cals	2g	7g (2g saturates)	38g (22g total sugars)	2g
CARDAMOM + PISTACHIO SHORTBREAD	315 cals	4g	13g (3g saturates)	44g (20g total sugars)	2g

INDEX

MICHAEL JOSEPH

UK | USA | Canada | Ireland | Australia
India | New Zealand | South Africa

Michael Joseph is part of the Penguin
Random House group of companies
whose addresses can be found at
global.penguinrandomhouse.com

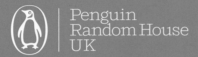

First published in Great Britain by
Michael Joseph, 2020
001

Text copyright © So Vegan, 2020
Photography copyright © Dan Jones, 2020

The moral right of the authors has been
asserted

Set in Franklin Gothic and Oswald

Colour reproduction by Altaimage Ltd
Printed and bound by Livonia Print, Latvia

A CIP catalogue record for this book is
available from the British Library

ISBN: 978–0–241–44871–7

www.greenpenguin.co.uk

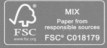